21-DAY ARTHRITIS DIET PLAN

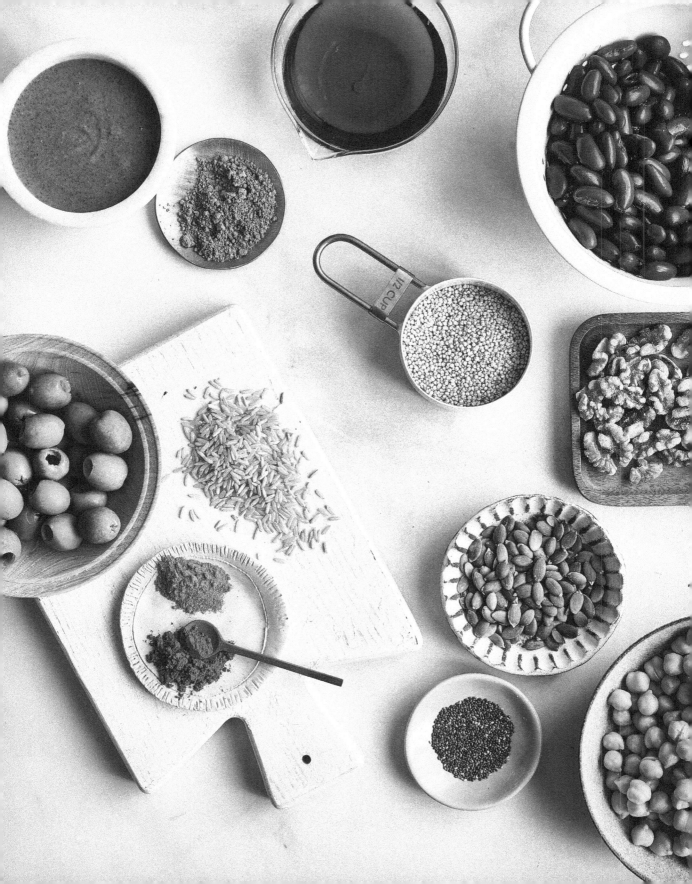

21-DAY
ARTHRITIS
DIET PLAN

Nutrition Guide and Recipes to Fight Osteoarthritis Pain and Inflammation

ANA REISDORF, MS, RD

PHOTOGRAPHY BY HELENE DUJARDIN

ROCKRIDGE
PRESS

Interior & Cover Designer: Diana Haas
Art Producer: Sara Feinstein
Editor: Mo Mozuch
Production Editor: Rachel Taenzler
Photography © 2020 Helene Dujardin
Food styling by Anna Hampton
Author photo courtesy of © Rachael Black Photography

ISBN: Print 978-1-64611-829-8 | eBook 978-1-64611-830-4
R0

To all my incredible registered dietitian
nutritionist colleagues who have supported my
career dreams and aspirations

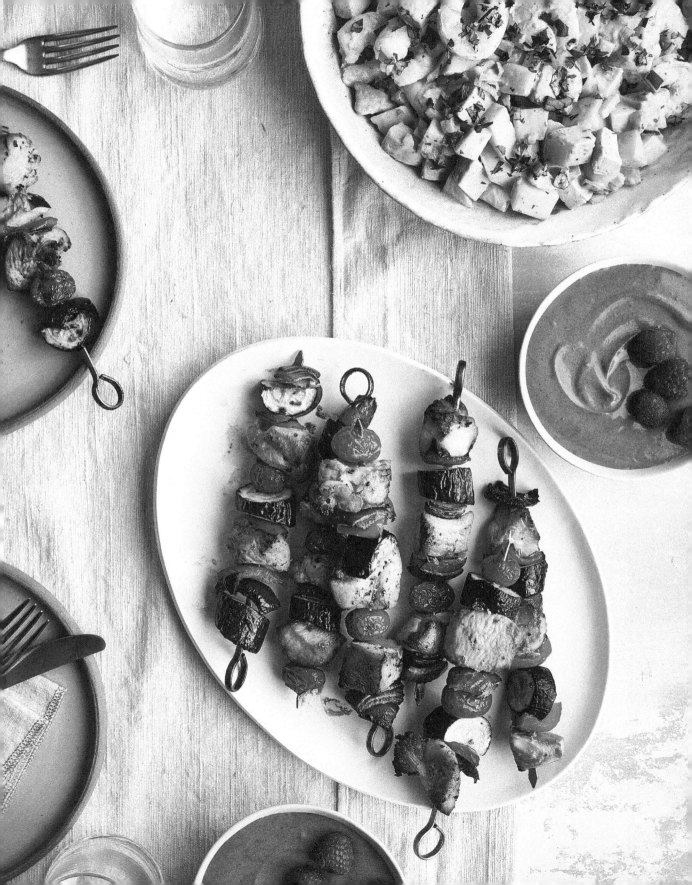

CONTENTS

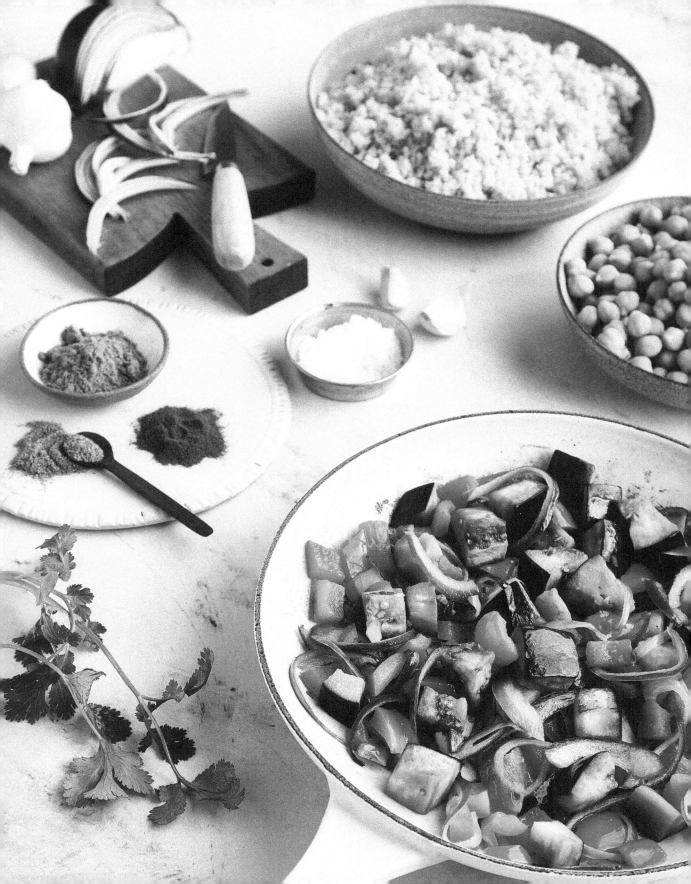

INTRODUCTION

WHEN I FIRST STARTED MY career in nutrition, all I wanted to do was help people lose weight. I was passionate about fitness and healthy eating and couldn't wait to share my knowledge with others.

My first job in health education focused on helping people prepare for weight-loss surgery. In this particular program, the patients were required to lose a certain amount of weight before surgery to help them start practicing the lifestyle changes that would be required after surgery. It also helped improve surgical outcomes by reducing blood pressure and blood sugar.

As a brand-new registered dietitian nutritionist, I was incredibly motivated to help my patients lose weight. On the first day of class, I showed up with an exercise video in hand. I was determined to make them walk off those pounds while we learned about healthy eating.

But I didn't realize the challenges I would face in trying to get my patients to move more. Not because they didn't want to exercise, but because they simply couldn't. I was naive about the amount of pain they were experiencing. For many, any significant exercise (especially walking) was completely out of the question due to a combination of excess body weight and arthritis pain.

In working with these patients over the next two years, I started to understand the vicious cycle this created. Arthritis pain led to lack of exercise, which led to weight gain. Excessive weight and increased arthritis pain made them even more sedentary.

I will admit, it was difficult for them to break the cycle. Weight-loss surgery was one possible solution to help get excess weight off and reduce their pain levels. But the surgery was six months away for these patients. And they were in pain now! They needed something to help them right away so they could start exercising more and lose the weight required for surgery.

I was determined to help them break the cycle and get their lives back. I knew the power of healthy food and the impact it could have on reducing pain and inflammation. I couldn't "cure" their pain, but I could help at least make it a little more manageable.

For this group of patients, I began to help them implement the principles of a healthy, anti-inflammatory diet, which are presented in this book. I taught them the power of fruits and vegetables, omega-3 fats, and anti-inflammatory herbs and spices. I encouraged them to get rid of foods that were causing pain and recommended pain-reducing foods to replace them with. I provided healthy meal plans and recipes so they could start to learn how to prepare the foods that were best for them.

I can't say they were all pain-free after six months. But several of them never needed weight-loss surgery because they were able to lose the weight they needed just by changing their diets. Some were able to reduce their pain to a point where exercise became fun again. Others were able to have necessary knee- or hip-replacement surgeries sooner than anticipated because they had lost enough weight to do so.

The diet presented in this book is not a weight-loss diet. It is an inflammation- and pain-reduction diet. Once these issues are under control, you may find yourself more motivated to exercise and continue to eat in a healthy manner, helping your body reach the optimal weight for you. The goal is to help you live the active, full life you deserve.

ABOUT THIS DIET

THE DIET PRESENTED IN THIS book is based on the principles of the Mediterranean diet, one of the healthiest diets on the planet. It is meant to give people struggling with osteoarthritis pain an evidence-based way to eat to reduce inflammation and help them live better with this chronic condition.

The diet emphasizes eating plenty of plant foods, although it is not a vegetarian diet. It does include both plant and animal sources of protein. It is also focused on healthy fats, like omega-3s and monounsaturated fats. This book provides recipes that can be modified to fit many eating preferences, if necessary.

In this book, you will find a 21-day meal plan that is delicious and easy to follow. My goal is not for you to follow it exactly, but to give you ideas for how you can start to eat in a healthier way and improve symptoms quickly.

It is important to note that managing osteoarthritis is not just about diet. Although food is powerful, it does not provide a cure for this disease. To truly reduce pain and improve symptoms a multifaceted approach is necessary. Other lifestyle changes, such as good sleep and the right amount of exercise, play a major role as well. Traditional medical treatment may be necessary to further reduce your pain, depending on the progression of the disease.

I want to give you a starting point by providing a few simple steps toward the pain-free life you want.

This book is not intended as a substitute for medical advice or to provide a "cure" for osteoarthritis. Any lifestyle changes, including diet, should always be discussed with a medical doctor.

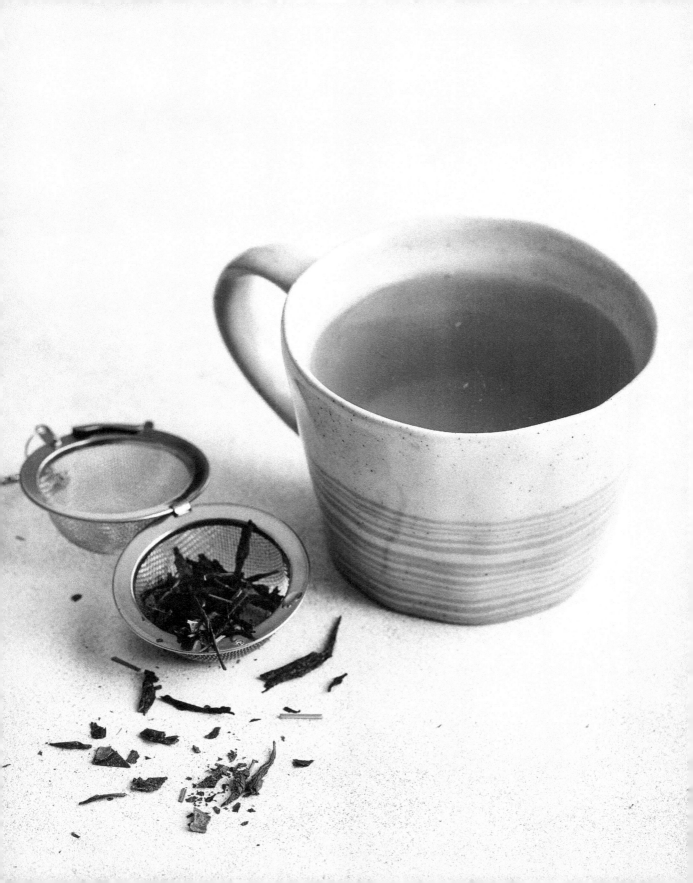

CHAPTER 1

Osteoarthritis Explained

THERE ARE OVER 100 DIFFERENT types of arthritis. Osteoarthritis (OA) is the most common: It impacts over 30 million adults in the United States, according to the Centers for Disease Control and Prevention (CDC).

Lifestyle and diet play a major role in helping manage the pain and inflammation associated with osteoarthritis. But in order to understand how to improve your symptoms, it is important to discuss the basics of this common joint disease.

This section will review the cause, progression, severity, and common treatments of osteoarthritis. The goal is for you to have an understanding of arthritis so you can take action toward improving your symptoms.

What Is Osteoarthritis?

Osteoarthritis is an inflammatory condition of the joints. A joint is anywhere that bones come together, such as the knees, hips, or fingers. The end of each bone is covered with a layer of protective tissue called cartilage. In OA patients, the cartilage breaks down. This leads to pain, lack of mobility, stiffness, swelling, and other symptoms. Due to the constant friction, osteoarthritis causes extremely painful bone spurs, or projections of bone along the edges of a bone, to develop.

The breakdown of cartilage seen in OA is primarily caused by wear and tear and damage to the joints over time. Therefore, this condition mainly occurs in older adults, although it can happen to younger people. It can develop in any joint that has been damaged or overused. OA is most common in the hips, knees, lower back, neck, hands, and feet.

Although the symptoms may be similar, OA is different from another common form of arthritis called rheumatoid arthritis (RA). RA is an auto-immune disorder that can lead to similar destruction of cartilage in the joints. But in RA, the cartilage damage occurs when the body attacks itself, not from wear and tear on the joints. Yet, many of the symptoms are similar.

Women are more likely to have arthritis than men. From 2013 to 2015, 26 percent of women and 19.1 percent of men in the United States reported ever having been diagnosed with arthritis, according to the CDC. However, the Arthritis Foundation reports that in people under 45 years old, men are more likely to have OA.

The CDC reports the prevalence for all types of arthritis by age. These are:

- Ages 18 to 44: 7.1 percent

- Ages 45 to 64: 29.3 percent

- Ages 65 or older: 49.6 percent

With such high rates of OA in the United States, it is probably no surprise that it is a leading cause of disability. Fortunately, medical treatment and lifestyle changes can help people manage their symptoms.

What Causes Osteoarthritis?

It was previously believed that osteoarthritis was simply a disease of damage to the joints caused by overuse. But the underlying cause of OA is not as simple as that. Although wear and tear does contribute to the progression of the disease, there are many different factors that may lead to developing OA.

The following are some of the most common causes of OA and how each contributes to the development of the disease.

HEREDITY

A family history of OA can increase your risk of developing the disease. People who have certain other diseases—including those that cause abnormal bone and cartilage growths as well as Paget's disease, which causes bone inflammation—are also more likely to develop OA, according to the Cleveland Clinic.

There are a few rare genetic defects that increase your risk of developing OA. One of these is a genetic mutation that affects the body's ability to produce collagen, a protein in cartilage. A person with this type of genetic abnormality may develop osteoarthritis as early as their 20s. Other genetic conditions that increase the risk for OA include defects in the way certain bones fit together, causing faster damage from wear and tear.

OBESITY

Being overweight puts pressure on the joints, particularly the knees and hips. The longer you are overweight, the more pressure is placed on the cartilage. It is no surprise that one of the major risk factors for OA is obesity.

But it's not just the knees and hips that are at greater risk for OA due to excess body weight. According to an article in *Annals of the Rheumatic Diseases*, being overweight increases the risk of hand OA as well, so there's more at play than just increased pressure on the joints. Additionally, it seems that losing excess pounds is not enough to improve symptoms: OA symptoms improve the most when body fat is lost.

One reason why obesity is linked with an increased risk of OA is that body fat produces proteins called adipokines, some of which play an important role in cartilage and bone maintenance and may also contribute to OA. Researchers know there is more to the connection between OA and excess body weight than simply pressure on the joints, but it is still not fully understood.

JOINT OVERUSE

OA can occur in joints that are overused, particularly those that are involved in repetitive movements like running or lifting heavy objects. Certain types of athletes are particularly at risk for joint, cartilage, and ligament damage due to overuse. People who stand for long periods of time at work or who do the same task over and over can also be at risk for cartilage damage.

Cartilage is meant to protect the joints from friction, but it can become trapped in a cycle of swelling when tissues in the joints are damaged. To repair joint tissues, the body releases certain chemicals that trigger the production of cartilage components: collagen, a type of connective tissue, and proteoglycans, which increase the resilience of the tissue. This is similar to what happens when you get a blister on your foot that turns into a callus from walking in the wrong shoes for too long. The cartilage may thicken, swell, and start to develop cracks. Eventually, the cartilage becomes damaged and rough and starts to break down. It can no longer properly and smoothly absorb the impact on the bones. This is when the classic symptoms of OA such as swelling, pain, and stiffness start to occur.

INJURIES

OA caused by injury is referred to as "post-traumatic arthritis." This is caused by a physical injury to the joint that leads to damage to the cartilage. According to the Cleveland Clinic, 12 percent of people with OA of the knee, hip, or ankle have post-traumatic arthritis triggered by some sort of injury.

The injury that leads to arthritis can vary but is usually from sports, a physical accident, or other trauma to the joint. The injury can damage the cartilage directly or change the joint so that the cartilage gets damaged more quickly. It is important to note that injury to the joint will not always result in OA, and that other factors such as body weight and genetic predisposition also play a role.

If you have had an injury to a specific joint, it is important to be evaluated by a doctor.

There are also a few other less common factors that may contribute to OA. Those with rheumatoid arthritis are more likely to develop OA. Hemochromatosis, a rare disorder related to iron absorption, also increases the risk. Acromegaly, a disorder that results from excessive levels of growth hormone, also impacts cartilage and bone health and may lead to OA.

What Are the Stages of Osteoarthritis?

Pain in your joints may lead you to see your doctor to get some relief. They may conduct a physical exam to evaluate the affected joints for flexibility, redness, swelling, and tenderness. This physical examination is the first step to diagnosing OA.

Depending on the findings of this exam, your doctor may recommend imaging tests such as X-rays or MRIs. An X-ray can show a doctor how much space there is between the bones and help them identify bone spurs. An MRI can produce an image of the bone, cartilage, and other soft tissues so they can evaluate the amount of damage, especially in more advanced cases.

Lab tests or a joint fluid analysis may be ordered to rule out RA and other similar conditions. Joint fluid can be tested for inflammatory markers, infection, and gout to make sure there aren't other underlying issues.

All these tests can help your doctor identify the stage of OA you are in. This is important to help the doctor determine your treatment options and begin to take the proper steps to slow down the progression of the disease. Here are the four stages of OA and the symptoms that occur at each stage:

STAGE 1

Stage 1 is when bone spur growth begins, but it is minor at this stage. Bone spurs are growths that develop where the bones connect once the cartilage in the joint is damaged. Most people do not experience significant pain at this stage, therefore they don't know they even have OA, unless they really over-extend themselves physically.

At this initial stage, your doctor may not recommend any specific treatment. You likely don't need any pain medications at this point. But preventative measures may stop the OA from getting worse. Losing weight, changing your diet, and strengthening the muscles around the joints can help. Certain supplements, such as glucosamine, chondroitin, and omega-3 fatty acids may also protect the joints from further damage and reduce inflammation.

STAGE 2

Stage 2 is considered "mild" OA. At this point, you may have larger bone spurs, and your cartilage is breaking down, but the amount of cartilage and space between the bones is still normal. Joint motion is also normal.

The bones are not rubbing together at stage 2, therefore you may not experience extreme pain. But after a lot of exercise, such as a day spent walking, you may start to feel joint stiffness and tenderness.

ARTHRITIS MEDICATIONS AND SIDE EFFECTS

The main symptom of OA is pain and discomfort. There are several medications that can be used to help manage pain. When you're using medications, it's even more important to discuss changes in your diet with your doctor. Many of these medications have side effects, particularly if you use them long-term, so it is important to always discuss your options with your physician. Here are the most commonly used medications for OA:

Analgesics are pain medications that reduce pain by blocking pain signals in the body. They do not reduce inflammation, which is frequently the underlying cause of pain. Tylenol, or acetaminophen, is a common type of analgesic.

Acetaminophen has many potential side effects, particularly at high doses. The most concerning is liver failure. Of the liver failure cases in the United States, around 40 percent are believed to be caused by acetaminophen toxicity. It can also cause gastrointestinal bleeds. The maximum daily dosage according to the US Food and Drug Administration (FDA) is 4,000 milligrams per day, so it is important to be aware of the total amount of this medication you are taking.

Topical analgesics are pain-relieving medications that are applied directly to the affected joint via ointments, creams, gels, or patches. They are available both over the counter and via prescription. Many are meant to provide immediate, short-term relief and may have to be reapplied regularly. Others may provide longer-term relief from inflammation and pain.

Common topical analgesics include: capsaicin, menthol, lidocaine patch, and trolamine salicylate. The main side effects of these medications are skin irritation, burning, or stinging at the affected area. Severe side effects, such as allergic reactions, are rare but should be reported to your doctor right away.

Nonsteroidal anti-inflammatory drugs (NSAIDs) are medications that reduce inflammation and pain. These are often effective for people with OA because they manage symptoms and may help prevent joint damage. They are also non-sedating, so they won't affect your mental function or make you feel drowsy.

There are many over-the-counter NSAIDs available, including ibuprofen, aspirin, diclofenac, and naproxen. There are also multiple options for prescription NSAIDs, depending on your specific condition. These medications can have side effects such as stomach bleeding, ulcers, and kidney problems, particularly if they are used for an extended period of time.

Corticosteroids (steroids) are extremely effective medications that are used short term to manage extreme flare-ups and quickly decrease inflammation and pain. They can be taken orally or injected directly into the joints. Common steroid medications are prednisone, hydrocortisone, and betamethasone.

But steroids have many potential side effects and are usually not recommended for long-term pain management. They can cause cataracts, blood sugar problems, and bone loss if taken for a long time.

Opioids are prescription pain medications that alter the way you feel pain but don't reduce inflammation. Common opioids include codeine, hydrocodone, fentanyl, and morphine.

These medications can be very effective for pain management, but they are habit-forming. They are usually prescribed when the patient is recovering from surgery or when severe pain management is required due to stage 4 OA.

Opioids can cause constipation or other digestive discomforts. They can lead to depression. They may also cause breathing problems during sleep, or make you feel drowsy or off-balance. Opioids should not be used with alcohol or other drugs, as these can make these side effects worse.

At this stage, getting the right diagnosis to take steps toward prevention is critical. Your doctor can help you develop a plan to prevent the OA from getting worse. The same measures that worked in stage 1 can also help in stage 2, such as losing weight, proper exercise, strength training, and a healthy diet.

Wearing the right shoes and practicing proper alignment when moving can help as well. If the OA is in the knee, a knee brace or a wrap worn during physical activity to stabilize the joint can help prevent further damage.

STAGE 3

Stage 3 is called "moderate" OA. This is when the damage to the cartilage can be seen in an MRI and the space between the bones starts to narrow. Most people with stage 3 OA begin to experience regular pain and swelling with most movement. This is when you may have joint stiffness in the morning or after sitting for an extended period of time.

Non-drug treatments, like weight loss, diet, and strength training, can still help at this point, but most people also need some type of pain management medication. Your doctor may recommend a cortisone shot three to four times a year to the affected joint to reduce inflammation and pain.

Oral pain medications such as NSAIDs, acetaminophen, or even narcotic medications may be required at this stage. These drugs have side effects and some have addictive potential, so it is important to discuss your pain management options with your doctor and understand what you are taking.

STAGE 4

Stage 4 is "severe" OA. People in this stage experience severe pain with any movement, making day-to-day activities such as walking very difficult. At this point, some or all of the cartilage between the joints is completely gone, and the joint is extremely stiff and almost immobile. There is little synovial fluid left to help reduce friction between the bones.

One of the treatment options for severe OA is surgery of the joint called bone realignment surgery. This is when the surgeon cuts the bone to change its alignment and prevent the bones from rubbing together. The surgery helps relieve pressure on the joints by moving the point of contact away from the part that has been the most damaged. Usually this type of surgery is most successful in younger patients.

Another surgical option is a joint replacement. This is usually the last resort to help relieve pain. A surgeon replaces the joint with a metal or plastic device. This type of surgery requires weeks or months to recover from and carries the risk of multiple complications. Additionally, a joint replacement can't guarantee you will not continue to have pain, and it may need to be redone.

The Diet-Arthritis Connection

Symptoms of osteoarthritis are caused by damage to the joints and the inflammation that results from this damage. Your diet cannot replace the cartilage in the joints or reverse the damage, but diet can help manage the inflammation and reduce pain.

Certain foods have anti-inflammatory abilities, while others can make inflammation worse. Inflammation is the body's reaction to physical or psychological stress. The inflammatory reaction is how the immune system tries to help the body heal. When there is an acute problem, like an infection or an injury, the immune system acts quickly to fight the irritant through inflammation that contains the damaged area. The body releases inflammatory proteins called cytokines, which alert the rest of the immune system that there is a problem.

But when there is a chronic problem like joint damage, the immune system is constantly triggering the inflammatory response. This leads to further joint damage and pain.

Cytokines and other inflammatory markers can also be triggered by certain foods. Foods like sugar and saturated fat can trigger the release of these inflammatory chemicals, whereas other foods with anti-inflammatory properties can calm the inflammatory response. Foods high in vitamins, minerals, certain fats, and antioxidants all have the ability to reduce inflammation and prevent further damage to the joints.

Additionally, a healthy diet can help with weight management. Excess body fat initiates the release of inflammatory cytokines, making pain worse. Every pound of excess weight puts four additional pounds of pressure on the joints. Maintaining a healthy weight can help slow the progression of OA.

Below is a list of foods to avoid and foods to include for managing the progression of OA. Many of these might be obvious: For example, you know that processed foods high in sugar are not beneficial. Foods to avoid include those high in sugar, salt, refined carbohydrates, and saturated fat, all of which trigger inflammation. The recommended foods have anti-inflammatory properties, are high in nutrients, and may help reduce pain.

Although shifting your way of eating may be a challenge at first, focusing on the overall benefit to your health and the potential to reduce the pain in your joints can help you work toward positive lifestyle changes.

FOODS TO INCLUDE

- **Proteins low in saturated fat:** lean red meat, poultry, or lamb

- **Oily fish high in omega-3 fatty acids:** salmon, mackerel, herring, sardines

- **Legumes and beans**

- **Nuts and seeds high in omega-3s:** chia, flaxseed, walnuts

- **Monounsaturated oils:** olive, avocado, and grapeseed oil

- **Fruits and vegetables:** especially green leafy vegetables and berries high in antioxidants

- **Whole grains:** oats, quinoa, millet, brown rice

- **Anti-inflammatory herbs and spices:** garlic, turmeric, ginger, cumin, etc.

- **Green tea**

- **Low fat dairy***

- **Gluten-containing grains****

FOODS TO AVOID

- **Foods high in sugar:** candy, pies, cookies, cakes, pastries

- **Sugar-sweetened beverages:** soda, fruit juice, sweet coffee drinks, sweet tea

- **Foods high in saturated fat:** processed meats, fatty cuts of meat, cheese

- **Refined carbohydrates:** white bread, regular pasta, chips, crackers, white rice

*Dairy has been shown to help with weight loss and muscle building, but it can be inflammatory for some people. We did not exclude dairy in the recipes in this book, but you can choose to prepare your food with nondairy alternatives.

**Gluten-containing grains can be inflammatory for those who are sensitive to them. We did not exclude whole grains in the recipes, but you can always substitute the gluten-containing grains for gluten-free options.

HOW TO GET A GOOD NIGHT'S SLEEP

The pain and stiffness from arthritis can contribute to difficulty sleeping. A 2018 study published in *BMC Musculoskeletal Disorders* found that more than half the study participants who had OA also had a sleep disorder.

Frequently, symptoms can be worse at night after the demands of the day are done. There is less stimulation at night, so there is nothing to distract you from the pain, making sleep difficult. Poor sleep is a trigger for inflammation, which will also exacerbate pain. The lack of sleep makes you tired, which triggers more inflammation and pain and causes more lack of sleep. It can be difficult to break this cycle.

Lack of sleep doesn't only make you tired. It can contribute to weight gain, which means even more pressure on the joints. The body and the mind need a good night's rest every night to function at their healthiest level.

Here are a few tips for getting a good night's sleep:

- **Stretch before bed.** Doing a few light stretches can help alleviate some muscle soreness and tension. Consider asking your doctor or a physical therapist for an appropriate stretching routine based on your particular pain areas.

- **Exercise regularly.** Physical activity helps promote a good night's rest. Aim to do any type of physical activity that you are able for at least 30 minutes a day. Swimming is a great exercise that takes pressure off the joints.

- **Use a heating pad.** Heat before bed can reduce inflammation and help muscles relax.

- **Practice meditation or deep breathing before bed.** Clearing your mind can help the body relax and reduce pain.

- **Invest in a quality mattress, bedding, and pillows.** You spend a third of your life in bed, so you need to make it comfortable, especially if you are already in pain. When shopping for a mattress, take your time to try them out at the store or consider shopping with companies that offer money-back guarantees. You can also ask your physical therapist for advice on the best type of mattress for you.

- **While sleeping, wedge a pillow between your legs for hip or knee pain.** Removing some of the pressure on these joints can help ease pain at night.

- **Take a magnesium or melatonin supplement.** These supplements or a calming tea like chamomile can promote relaxation at bedtime and help you get a good night's sleep. Be careful with magnesium, as it can cause diarrhea in higher doses, so start slowly.

- **Go to bed and wake up at the same time every day.** The body likes predictability. If you go to bed at the same time, your body will automatically start to relax before bedtime.

- **Have a bedtime routine.** A regular bedtime routine signals to your body to relax and fall asleep at a specific time. This routine can involve many things, like taking a warm bath, reading a calming book, or enjoying a warm cup of herbal tea. No matter what activities you choose, the important thing is to do them consistently. This way your body and mind receive the signal that it is time to go to bed.

- **Speak to your doctor about medication.** A sleeping aid may help you relax and break the fatigue-pain cycle.

If you are not sleeping well, this will influence every other aspect of your life. So, prioritize a good night's sleep and implement some of the steps outlined previously to help you get there.

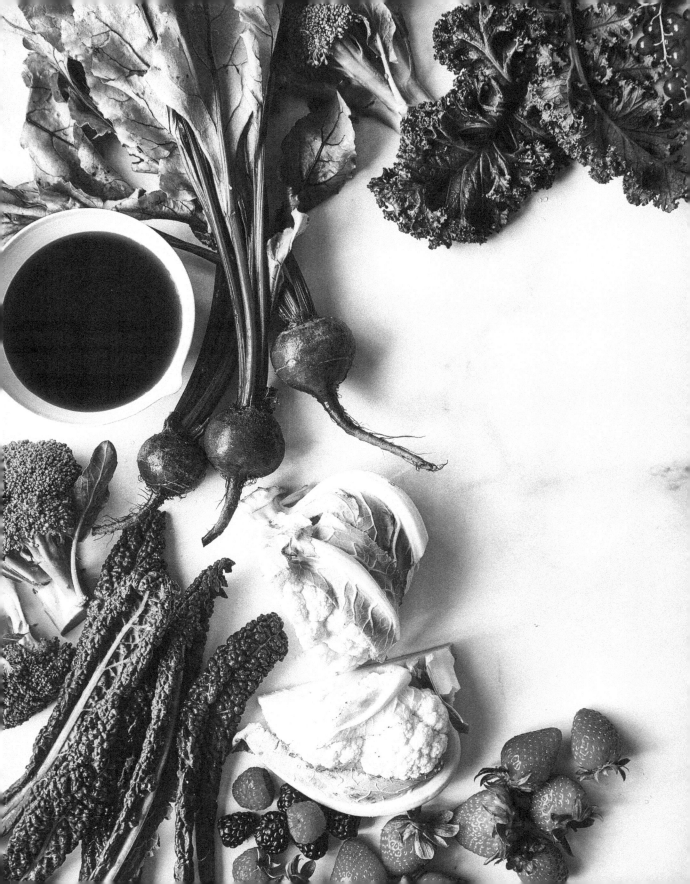

CHAPTER 2

Arthritis & Nutrition

WHEN YOU ARE IN PAIN, you want immediate relief. Diet is an easy place to start making lifestyle changes to improve your OA symptoms. If you have ever searched online for diet advice for OA, you may have felt overwhelmed. There is a lot of advice out there about what you should and shouldn't eat.

In this chapter, I will discuss the connection between your nutrition and your arthritis. This includes highlighting specific nutrients and plant compounds that have shown particular promise in helping improve symptoms of OA by reducing inflammation and pain.

The goal at the end of this chapter is to leave you with a straightforward, research-driven strategy to build a healthier kitchen from refrigerator to pantry. The information provided here, in combination with the meal plan and recipes, will give you a specific road map to follow toward a healthier diet for OA.

What Makes Healthy Food So Healthy?

What makes a food healthy or unhealthy? In general, it is the vitamins, minerals, fats, or other compounds that promote health. The following are some powerful ingredients, found in different foods, that contribute to a reduction in inflammation and support overall joint health.

Many of the nutrients listed in this section are plant chemicals called phytonutrients, which have anti-inflammatory and antioxidant properties. Phytonutrients contribute to the vibrant colors, tastes, and smells of plants.

Humans who eat fruits and vegetables high in phytonutrients can benefit from their protective abilities. Phytonutrients help repair damaged DNA, help with detoxification, fight oxidative stress, and support healthy joints.

ANTHOCYANINS

Anthocyanins are phytonutrients that give certain fruits and vegetables, like eggplant or raspberries, their purple or red color. Recent research shows their anti-inflammatory properties can reduce arthritis symptoms.

A 2017 study published in *Nutrients* evaluated the impact of strawberries, which are rich in anthocyanins, on the symptoms of osteoarthritis. Seventeen subjects with OA were given either 50 grams per day of freeze-dried strawberries or a placebo for 12 weeks. During the study period, various inflammation markers were evaluated as well as pain scores and quality of life assessments.

At the end of 12 weeks, markers of inflammation and cartilage degradation were significantly improved in the strawberry group. Subjects also reported decreases in pain while consuming the strawberries.

COLLAGEN

Collagen is the most abundant protein in the body and the main protein found in cartilage. Supplementing your diet with collagen may help the body repair damaged cartilage and support joint health in OA.

A 2006 review published in *Current Medical Research and Opinion* evaluated the available clinical studies on collagen supplements for OA. They found that collagen supplements are well absorbed and could help improve pain and joint function.

DIALLYL DISULFIDE

Diallyl disulfide (DADS) is a sulfur-based compound found in foods in the allium family, such as garlic and onions. It contributes to the strong odor and flavor of these foods.

A 2017 lab study published in the *Journal of Cellular Biochemistry* evaluated the protective effects of DADS against oxidative stress and cell breakdown in chondrocytes, or cartilage-producing cells. The addition of DADS was found to significantly influence the chondrocytes, and the study concluded that DADS could be a natural way to protect cartilage.

A 2009 study in *Osteoarthritis and Cartilage* found similar results, with a garlic sulfur compound being able to directly target inflammation in joint cells.

EPIGALLOCATECHIN GALLATE (EGCG)

Green tea contains a powerful anti-inflammatory polyphenol called epigallo-catechin gallate (EGCG).

A 2018 study published in *Clinical Nutrition* evaluated the impact of green tea on the symptoms of osteoarthritis of the knee. Fifty subjects received either a green tea extract combined with an NSAID medication called diclofenac or the diclofenac alone for four weeks. Subjects were evaluated for pain via multiple standard scales and asked about any adverse effects of the intervention.

There was no difference in stiffness between the groups, but subjects who received the green tea in combination with the medication reported significantly better physical function.

OLEOCANTHAL

An anti-inflammatory compound found in virgin olive oil called oleocanthal is one of the reasons why the Mediterranean diet is so beneficial for overall health and for osteoarthritis. Some studies have found that this compound may be as effective as ibuprofen, a common NSAID, for reducing inflammation.

Emerging research has found that oleocanthal works by targeting specific signaling proteins that trigger inflammation and cartilage destruction. It may also help control production of nitric oxide, a free radical that can harm the joints. So, not only does it help decrease pain, it may also help slow the progression of the disease altogether.

OMEGA-3

Omega-3 fatty acids are anti-inflammatory fats found in oily fish, walnuts, and flaxseeds.

A 2011 animal study published in *Osteoarthritis and Cartilage* evaluated the effect of a diet high in omega-3s on the development of OA. In this study

SUPPLEMENT ABCs

Using effective dietary supplements may be one way to add more nutrients to your regimen that you simply can't get from diet alone. The three below, which I like to call the "ABCs of osteoarthritis," can help relieve OA symptoms.

When choosing dietary supplements, always check if the product has been USP-verified or undergone other third-party testing for purity and quality. Remember that dietary supplements are not regulated by the FDA, so a good-quality brand will voluntarily test their products in other ways. Also, do not take dietary supplements without speaking to your physician first, particularly if you are already taking other medications.

- **Avocado-soybean unsaponifiables (ASU):** An ASU is an extract made from one-third avocado oil and two-thirds soybean oil, this anti-inflammatory oil actively fights the inflammation and joint destruction seen in OA. It also promotes cartilage repair through the stimulation of new collagen.

  A 2008 meta-analysis published in *Osteoarthritis and Cartilage* that involved 664 subjects with OA found that ASU was able to reduce pain. The recommended dose is one 300 milligram softgel daily.

- **Boswellic acid (Indian frankincense):** This is a resin from the *Boswellia serrata* tree, native to India. It has been found to reduce symptoms of OA through its pain-reducing, anti-inflammatory properties. It may also help slow cartilage loss.

  A 2008 study published in *Arthritis Research & Therapy* found that supplementing with 100 to 250 milligrams of boswellic acid each day could improve function and pain within a week. After three months, there were indications that it was starting to help slow cartilage damage.

- **Curcumin:** This anti-inflammatory is a component of turmeric, a yellow-colored Asian spice. A 2010 clinical trial published in *Alternative Medicine Review* found that a turmeric supplement helped significantly reduce pain and improve joint function in 100 patients with knee OA.

    Although adding turmeric to food is beneficial and delicious, a supplement is recommended in order to get a concentrated and effective dose for pain reduction, as curcumin only makes up around 3 percent of the turmeric spice. The recommended dose for capsules is 400 to 600 milligrams three times a day.

researchers found that a diet rich in omega-3 fats slowed disease development and improved bone density.

However, it is important to note that a 2015 review on omega-3s and OA published in the *American Journal of Orthopedics* found that study results were inconsistent. Lab and animal research have consistently shown that omega-3s can reduce joint inflammation, but the results for humans won't be clear without further study.

QUERCETIN

Quercetin is an anti-inflammatory flavonoid that has been shown to reduce symptoms of osteoarthritis. It is found in many fruits and vegetables, such as green leafy vegetables, apples, and red onions.

A study published in *Bioscience, Biotechnology, and Biochemistry* evaluated the use of a dietary supplement that included a combination of quercetin, glucosamine, and chondroitin on the symptoms of OA. Glucosamine and chondroitin are components of cartilage commonly found in joint supplements. Forty-six OA patients were given the combination supplement for three months. Subjects had significantly improved synovial fluid (fluid in the joints that reduces friction), decreased pain, and improved ability to perform daily activities while taking this combination supplement.

SULFORAPHANE

Sulforaphane is a natural antioxidant found in cruciferous vegetables such as Brussels sprouts, cabbage, and broccoli. It has been shown to slow the degeneration of cartilage, which means the earlier you start increasing your intake, the better.

A 2013 study published in *Arthritis & Rheumatology* found that sulforaphane actively slowed disease progression and cartilage damage in mice with OA. Researchers found that this compound was able to directly block enzymes that lead to joint destruction. It can also help reduce inflammation in the joints and possibly decrease pain and swelling.

Superfoods

The focus of the recipes in this book is to include as many "superfoods" as possible. Although there is no formal definition of the term "superfood," it is generally accepted that in order for a food to be called "super," it must have few unhealthy aspects while containing many health-supporting nutrients. The Mediterranean-style diet presented in this book is full of foods that are considered super healthy (and super tasty). Many are high in the nutrients we discussed in "What Makes Healthy Food So Healthy?" on page 15.

Here are a few foods in which you will find power nutrients for OA and for your overall health:

- **Broccoli:** This vegetable is incredibly high in the antioxidant sulforaphane. Other foods with this nutrient include Brussels sprouts, cabbage, bok choy, cauliflower, kale, watercress, and arugula.

- **Berries:** Raspberries, blueberries, cranberries, cherries, and strawberries should all be a regular part of your diet due to their high anthocyanin content. They are also an incredible source of fiber, vitamin C, and folate. They have been found to lower the risk of many chronic diseases from cancer to high cholesterol.

- **Beets:** The deep red color of beets is a sign that they are loaded with nutrients. They contain vitamins and antioxidants like folate, vitamin C, anthocyanin, iron, and nitrates. Betalain, a pigment in beets, has been found to help reduce OA pain.

- **Bone broth:** Bone broth is a nutrient-rich broth that results from boiling animal bones for 12 to 24 hours. This liquid is loaded with collagen and important joint-supporting minerals such as calcium and phosphorous. Bone broth is not the same as standard store-bought broth. But due to the popularity of bone broth for health, it is now easy to find real bone broth in most stores.

- **Olive oil:** Olive oil is not only high in the anti-inflammatory compound oleocanthal, it is also a great source of monounsaturated fat, which can help improve cholesterol levels and may help support a healthy immune system.

- **Fatty fish, like wild salmon:** Omega-3s are powerful anti-inflammatory fats. Most of us are lacking omega-3s in our diets due to not eating enough fish or other foods high in this healthy fat. Salmon, herring, mackerel, and sardines are all high in omega-3s.

- **Garlic:** Garlic and all the other vegetables in the allium family, such as onion and shallots, are high in two powerful nutrients called allicin and DADS. Allicin, in particular, has anti-inflammatory, antiviral, and anti-bacterial properties. The combination of these two nutrients makes garlic and other related foods "super."

- **Black currants:** These small berries are loaded with antioxidants. They have antimicrobial, antiviral, and antiseptic properties. They may promote heart health.

Adding these and many of the other superfoods included in the recipe section of this book will help boost the nutrient, antioxidant, and anti-inflammatory content of your diet.

Mediterranean Magic

The Mediterranean diet has consistently been called one of the healthiest diets in the world. It is based on the traditional nutrient-dense foods and incredible flavors found in countries along the Mediterranean Sea, such as Greece and Italy.

Scientific interest in the Mediterranean diet began in the 1950s and 1960s, when observational studies noted that there were lower rates of heart disease in this area of the world compared with the United States and Northern Europe. It was later discovered that one of the reasons for the lower rates of heart disease could be that the diet consumed in this region had powerful anti-inflammatory properties that were protective of the heart and could help reduce the risk of many other modern chronic diseases.

The Mediterranean diet is a plant-based diet, although it does not exclude animal products. It includes plant-based dishes with large amounts of vegetables, whole grains, fruit, legumes, nuts, and seeds. It includes small amounts of dairy products, particularly cheese and yogurt. The primary fat used for cooking

HOW TO BUY GOOD OLIVE OIL

Olive oil, with its anti-inflammatory properties, is one of the most important ingredients in this diet. It will be used in almost every recipe, from sautés to salad dressings. This is why it's important to shell out a few extra dollars for a high-quality brand. When it comes to purchasing olive oil, you really do get what you pay for.

When looking for an olive oil, always look for extra-virgin olive oil. "Light" or "first press" are terms that don't mean much, but extra-virgin olive oil contains the most naturally occurring nutrients. Double-check labels to make sure you aren't buying a blend full of safflower or grapeseed oil.

The term "product of" on the front of the bottle also doesn't mean anything, as it only indicates where the olive oil was bottled. Instead, look for a bottle that has the name of the estate where it was grown, pressed, and bottled.

Avoid oils that come in clear bottles, since light can damage the delicate anti-inflammatory compounds inside. Olive oil should ideally be used within 18 months of its harvest date, not its "use by" date, which is based on the time it was bottled. The fresher the better.

Be sure to store your olive oil properly. Do not store it near heat or a bright window, as these can destroy the delicate oil. Be cautious of how high you heat olive oil. It is not meant to be used for deep frying. It is best for lower-heat sautéing, drizzling, or salad dressings.

is olive oil, and the diet incorporates other monounsaturated fats such as olives, nuts, and avocados. The animal foods consumed include fish and poultry, with a limited intake of red meat. Overall, this is a flavorful, nutrient-rich diet full of vitamins, minerals, plant polyphenols, and antioxidants.

Another important piece of the Mediterranean diet is that it's focused on "slow" foods that take time to prepare. This means it is low in processed foods and sugar as well as highly inflammatory saturated and trans fats found in many of our modern convenience foods.

An important element of the Mediterranean diet is the emphasis on the lifestyle and community aspects of health. Traditionally, people in this area of the world are physically active throughout the day. Meals are prepared and enjoyed at a leisurely pace. They regularly share meals with family and friends while enjoying a glass of red wine. The Mediterranean diet truly offers a delicious and nutritious way to improve your health with food.

Your New Kitchen

Before you dive into your 21-day diet plan and recipes, you will have to do some restocking in your kitchen and pantry. Clear out foods that don't serve your health. Of course, many of the recipes require fresh ingredients, but you can start to gather various staples to make meal prep easier as you begin to make this diet a seamless part of your life.

The goal is to make this way of eating into a lifestyle. This means you will have to have the right ingredients on hand to help ensure that you are surrounded by the healthiest foods. If it is not easy or convenient, you aren't going to stick with it.

But success with any lifestyle change does require a little planning and preparation. Take a bit of time before you get started to review this new kitchen food list and hit the grocery store with the list in hand.

THE PANTRY

Stocking up on pantry staples is a great place to start your new healthy way of eating. Many pantry items keep for a long time, so you can always buy in bulk to save money. For some vegetables, like tomatoes, green beans, or artichokes,

I always like to keep canned options on hand for busy weeknights or for weeks when I don't have time to make it to the grocery store.

To keep the cost down, you don't have to buy all these items at once. Pick three to five recipes that use similar seasonings or ingredients and start with those. Eventually, you will have all the ingredients you need to make all the recipes in this book. The goal is not to break the bank, but to help you adopt a sustainable lifestyle to help you manage your OA symptoms.

Here are a few of the pantry staples you will see in the recipe section of the book:

- Quinoa
- Brown rice
- Rolled oats
- Whole-wheat bread
- Pasta (whole-wheat or gluten-free)
- Couscous
- High-quality extra-virgin olive oil
- Almond butter
- Canned beans (red beans, cannellini beans, chickpeas)
- Canned tomatoes
- Canned green beans

- Canned salmon
- Vegetable and chicken broth
- Canned artichokes
- Olives
- Matcha powder
- Chia seeds
- Stevia
- Pure maple syrup
- Soy sauce
- Cinnamon
- Walnuts
- Pepitas or pumpkin seeds

- Vanilla extract
- Turmeric
- Ground ginger
- Sriracha or other hot sauce
- Dried cranberries
- Bread crumbs (whole-wheat or gluten-free)
- Dijon mustard
- Red wine vinegar
- Balsamic vinegar
- Sea salt
- Black pepper

THE REFRIGERATOR

Although refrigerator items won't last as long as those in the pantry, there are still plenty of items you can keep on hand because they will be used often in recipes. But when eating a diet based on fresh fruits and vegetables, you may need to purchase produce a bit more often than you might be used to. This will likely mean going to the store at least once or twice a week.

I like to keep my meal planning simple because I hate throwing away unused fresh produce. I focus on two or three fresh vegetables and two or three fruits a week. I try not to buy too much. Although it is important to eat a variety of fruits and veggies, I vary them week to week rather than day to day. This helps me save money and prevents food waste. In the 21-day meal plan, the meals are paired together based on similar ingredients so you can follow the plan without a ton of wasted food.

But there are many refrigerator ingredients that you can stock up on that may last several weeks. Always check the "use by" date to ensure the freshest product. Here are a few with longer shelf-lives than produce that you'll be using again and again:

- Almond milk or other nondairy milk
- Plain and flavored Greek yogurt
- Unsalted butter
- Feta cheese
- Parmesan cheese
- Mozzarella cheese

- Eggs (large)
- Pesto
- Red potatoes
- Sweet potatoes
- Fresh ginger root
- Onions (white and red)

- Garlic
- Shallots
- Limes
- Oranges
- Lemon juice
- Tahini
- Hummus

THE FREEZER

The freezer is a meal prepper's best friend. You can prepare soups, stews, or casseroles ahead of time and freeze them for a quick defrost on busy week-nights. Many of the recipes in the book lend themselves well to being made ahead and frozen.

The freezer also allows you to keep a greater variety of vegetables, berries, and protein on hand that would otherwise go bad if not eaten quickly. Store-bought frozen fruits and vegetables may actually be more nutritious than fresh ones because they are frequently flash frozen immediately after they are

CONCENTRATE ON TART CHERRY JUICE

Tart cherries contain remarkable levels of anti-inflammatory properties. Their juice has been found to help reduce pain and inflammation in people with OA. The anthocyanins in tart cherries may also help maintain healthy collagen inside the joints.

A 2013 study published in *Osteoarthritis and Cartilage* evaluated the use of tart cherry juice in improving symptoms of OA. Forty-six patients were given either two 8-ounce bottles or a placebo daily for six weeks. They were evaluated for various pain and function scores, walking times, and inflammation. Function and pain scores improved after the cherry juice treatment. Most notably, inflammation was significantly reduced in the experimental group.

Many clinical studies use two 8-ounce doses of cherry juice in their research. But drinking 16 ounces of juice daily may not be cost-effective and can involve a significant amount of calories and sugar.

If you are looking to add tart cherry juice to your daily routine to help reduce inflammation, think about purchasing the concentrate or a tart cherry powder instead of the juice. Consider taking 1 ounce of the concentrate or 400 milligrams of the concentrated capsules to help improve your OA symptoms. You'll get the same health benefits at a fraction of the cost.

picked, preserving all the nutrients inside. Choose heartier fruits and veggies such as peas and corn to keep in the freezer, as these tend to defrost well.

Frozen fish is also generally more affordable than fresh fish, so you can add higher-quality varieties to your diet. With protein, just be sure to use safe defrosting methods by taking it out of the freezer and moving it into the refrigerator at least 24 to 48 hours before you plan on cooking. Do not leave food on the counter to defrost.

Here are a few items to keep in your freezer:

- Blueberries, strawberries, and blackberries
- Broccoli
- Cauliflower
- Asparagus
- Peas
- Corn
- Carrots
- Spiralized zucchini or other vegetables
- Vegetable mixes
- Whole-wheat bread
- Prepared grains such as quinoa, steel-cut oats, and brown rice
- Boneless, skinless chicken breasts
- Fish
- Shrimp
- Ground turkey

The Recipes

The Mediterranean-style diet and recipes presented in this book are not only healthy, they are also delicious. If a diet is not tasty, it will not be sustainable, no matter how healthy it is. These simple recipes were designed with flavor in mind to support you on your journey toward relieving your OA pain.

The recipes may include more fruits and vegetables than you are used to eating. But increasing your intake of plant foods high in anti-inflammatory phytochemicals is one of the best ways to decrease pain. These plant foods are balanced with protein, healthy fats, and whole grains to help you create well-rounded and delicious meals you can truly enjoy.

LABELS

Throughout the book, you will find the recipes labeled in various ways. These labels are meant to assist you in choosing the recipe that is best for your particular situation or lifestyle. A few of the labels that you will see in this book include:

- **Make Ahead:** Specifically designed for those who like to cook once and eat all week (or for a few days at least). If you choose to meal prep ahead, just remember the basics of food safety and reheating foods to the proper temperature, if that is required.

- **One Pot:** One-pot recipes are designed to reduce the post-meal cleanup and streamline your meal prep. They use either one pot or one sheet pan. They do not require special equipment to prepare.

- **Quick & Easy:** This recipe category is full of meals that take 30 minutes or less for busy weeknights when you have to get dinner on the table right away.

- **Leftovers Lunch:** A great way to save money and eat healthier is to pack your lunch. The recipes in this category keep well and can be enjoyed for lunch at work the following day.

TIPS

We also wanted to include a few tips, which will be used throughout the book to help you personalize the recipes provided:

- **Substitution Tip:** This will mention a potential recipe substitution for if you're missing ingredients or want added flavor, e.g., "For extra spice, substitute jalapeño peppers for red pepper."

- **Cooking Tip:** This will provide you with special preparation tips that don't fall under normal recipe instructions, e.g., "If you need avocados to ripen faster, place them in a paper bag for one to two days."

- **On the Menu:** Here, you'll find suggestions for serving your food or for pairing recipes in the book.

- **The Good Stuff:** This highlights an ingredient that is particularly beneficial for OA.

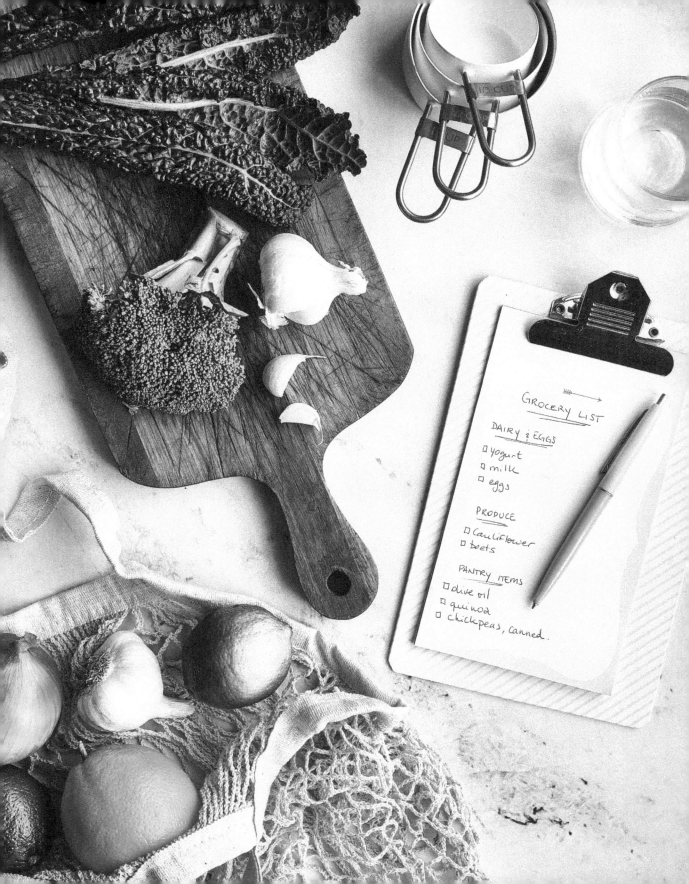

GROCERY LIST

DAIRY & EGGS

☐ yogurt
☐ milk
☐ eggs

PRODUCE

☐ cauliflower
☐ beets

PANTRY ITEMS

☐ olive oil
☐ quinoa
☐ chickpeas, canned.

CHAPTER 3

The 21-Day Arthritis Meal Plan

THE 21-DAY ARTHRITIS MEAL PLAN is designed to provide a template of how you can begin to implement the diet for OA discussed in chapter 2. The menu includes three weeks of meals with breakfast, lunch, dinner, and a snack. Although it is not a "weight-loss" diet, it is based on consuming 1,800 calories per day, which should result in moderate weight loss for most people. Remember, every pound of weight lost equals four pounds less pressure on your joints, so even shedding a few pounds can start to make a difference.

In order to make meal planning easier, the 21-day plan also includes a shopping list and tips for meal prep. The goal is to make it simple to follow, so you can begin to feel better as soon as possible.

Week 1

The first week is always the most challenging. It takes time to make a lifestyle change and adjust to a new way of eating. You will have to purchase and prepare foods that may be unfamiliar to you. You may need to plan meals and cook more than you are used to. This change will take effort and willpower as you learn a whole new way to eat and think about food.

Feel free to tailor the meal plan, mixing and matching days or individual meals. There is no need to follow the meal plan exactly as written, just make sure to update the shopping lists for each week.

The goal with this plan is to start to make sustainable long-term changes to the way you eat. Be patient with yourself. You don't need to be "perfect" every day, but it is important to focus on incremental progress. Making changes a little at a time is how you make these changes stick.

Week 1 Meal Plan

....

SUNDAY

Breakfast: 2 Make-Ahead Egg, Red Onion, and Brussels Sprout Breakfast "Muffins" (page 61)

Lunch: Crab Salad Sandwich (page 80)

Dinner: Lamb Chili (page 124)

Snack: Blueberry, Spinach, and Almond Butter Smoothie (page 54)

....

MONDAY

Breakfast: Blueberry, Spinach, and Almond Butter Smoothie (page 54) and 1 piece of whole-wheat toast with 1 teaspoon of butter

Lunch: Leftover Crab Salad Sandwich

Dinner: 6 ounces of rotisserie chicken, 1 baked sweet potato with 1 tablespoon butter, and Spinach and Strawberry Salad (page 72)

Snack: 1 apple topped with 1 tablespoon of almond butter

....

TUESDAY

Breakfast: 2 leftover Make-Ahead Egg, Red Onion, and Brussels Sprout Breakfast "Muffins" (page 61)

Lunch: Chopped Chicken Salad (page 76) on 2 slices whole-wheat bread and 1 apple

Dinner: Italian Burgers with Garlic Mayo and Red Onion Quick Pickle (page 116)

Snack: Frozen Yogurt with Mixed Berry Sauce (page 139)

WEDNESDAY

Breakfast: Overnight Oats with Dried Cranberries (page 59) and ⅓ cup of walnuts

Lunch: Leftover Italian Burgers with Garlic Mayo and Red Onion Quick Pickle

Dinner: Maple and Citrus–Glazed Salmon (page 103) and 1 baked sweet potato with 1 teaspoon of butter

Snack: ⅓ cup of dried cranberries and ⅓ cup of walnuts

THURSDAY

Breakfast: 2 leftover Make-Ahead Egg, Red Onion, and Brussels Sprout Breakfast "Muffins" (page 61)

Lunch: 8 ounces of leftover Maple and Citrus–Glazed Salmon mixed with 1 tablespoon mayonnaise on 1 whole-wheat hamburger bun

Dinner: Balsamic-Glazed Pork Tenderloin (page 120), Spinach and Strawberry Salad (page 72), 1 cup of brown rice

Snack: Frozen Yogurt with Mixed Berry Sauce (page 139)

FRIDAY

Breakfast: Overnight Oats with Dried Cranberries (page 59) and ⅓ cup of walnuts

Lunch: Leftover Lamb Chili

Dinner: Quick Tofu and Veggie Stir-Fry (page 92) and 1 cup of brown rice

Snack: ⅓ cup of dried cranberries and ⅓ cup of walnuts

SATURDAY

Breakfast: Mediterranean Breakfast Tostada (page 65) and 1 whole orange

Lunch: Leftover Quick Tofu and Veggie Stir-Fry and 1 cup of brown rice

Dinner: Orange Chicken and Quinoa Bowl (page 109)

Snack: 1 apple topped with 1 tablespoon of almond butter

WEEK 1 SHOPPING LIST

Don't be intimidated by the week 1 shopping list. Many of these items will be utilized throughout the entire 21-day plan. The basics are all covered here, so you won't have to purchase them again.

DAIRY AND EGGS

- ❑ Almond milk, 1 (½-gallon) carton
- ❑ Butter, or olive oil–based spread
- ❑ Cheese, crumbled feta, 2 (6-ounce) cartons
- ❑ Cheese, shredded Monterey Jack, 1 (8-ounce) bag
- ❑ Eggs, large, omega-3 fortified, 18
- ❑ Frozen yogurt, vanilla, 1 (16-ounce) carton
- ❑ Greek yogurt, plain, 2 (6-ounce) containers

CANNED AND BOTTLED ITEMS

- ❑ Almond butter, 1 jar
- ❑ Artichoke hearts, 1 (14-ounce) can
- ❑ Broth, low-sodium chicken, 2 (14-ounce) cans
- ❑ Cannellini beans, 1 (14-ounce) can
- ❑ Dijon mustard, 1 (16-ounce) jar
- ❑ Hot sauce, like sriracha
- ❑ Kidney beans, low-sodium, 3 (14-ounce) cans
- ❑ Maple syrup or honey
- ❑ Nonstick cooking spray, 1 bottle
- ❑ Olive oil, extra-virgin, 1 (32-ounce) bottle
- ❑ Olive oil mayonnaise
- ❑ Olives, black, sliced and pitted, 1 (2.25-ounce) can
- ❑ Sesame oil, 1 (5-ounce) bottle
- ❑ Soy sauce, low-sodium, 1 (16-ounce) bottle
- ❑ Tomatoes, crushed, 2 (14-ounce) cans
- ❑ Vinegar, apple cider, 1 (16-ounce) bottle
- ❑ Vinegar, balsamic, 1 (16-ounce) bottle
- ❑ Vinegar, red wine, 1 (16-ounce) bottle

FROZEN FOODS

- ❑ Blackberries, frozen (16 ounces)
- ❑ Blueberries, frozen (16 ounces)
- ❑ Raspberries, frozen (8 ounces)
- ❑ Strawberries, frozen (8 ounces)
- ❑ Optional: substitute 3 (16-ounce) bags of frozen mixed berries

PANTRY ITEMS

- ❑ Black pepper
- ❑ Bread, whole-wheat
- ❑ Bread crumbs
- ❑ Cayenne pepper
- ❑ Chia seeds
- ❑ Chili powder
- ❑ Cornstarch
- ❑ Cranberries, dried
- ❑ Cumin, dried
- ❑ Garlic powder
- ❑ Hamburger buns, whole-wheat
- ❑ Italian herbs, dried
- ❑ Matcha powder
- ❑ Oregano, dried
- ❑ Quinoa
- ❑ Red pepper flakes
- ❑ Rice, brown
- ❑ Rolled oats, 1 (42-ounce) container
- ❑ Sage, dried
- ❑ Sea salt
- ❑ Tortillas, corn
- ❑ Walnuts, chopped, 1 (1-pound) bag

PRODUCE

- ❑ Apples (3)
- ❑ Baby spinach, 1 large bag
- ❑ Bell peppers, red (4)
- ❑ Broccoli florets (2 cups)
- ❑ Brussels sprouts (2 cups)
- ❑ Cilantro, fresh (1 bunch)
- ❑ Dill, fresh (1 package)
- ❑ Garlic (2 heads)
- ❑ Ginger root, medium (2)
- ❑ Kale, 1 bag, chopped
- ❑ Lemons (2)
- ❑ Lime (1)
- ❑ Mushrooms, shiitake, 2 containers
- ❑ Onions, green (1 bunch)
- ❑ Onions, red (5)

WEEK 1 TIPS

The goal of this 21-day plan is not to spend the next three weeks in the kitchen. The plan is designed so that there are many meals that utilize leftovers or that can be prepped once and eaten multiple times.

Look for ways to save time in the kitchen by meal prepping or using convenience foods. Purchase pre-cut vegetables when possible—they may be especially useful if your OA is in your hands. Spend a bit of time on Sunday washing and chopping your vegetables ahead of time. Put your fruit, like the apples and oranges, on the counter so they are front and center when you want to grab a snack.

A few of the meals to make ahead include the Crab Salad Sandwiches, Overnight Oats with Dried Cranberries, and Make-Ahead Egg, Red Onion, and Brussels Sprout Breakfast "Muffins," all of which you can eat for two meals. Many of the lunches also utilize leftovers from the night before. Two meals use store-bought rotisserie chicken to reduce cooking even further. Make Tuesday's Chopped Chicken Salad on Monday night with the leftovers. You can prep it while your sweet potato bakes. If you did your veggie prep on Sunday, your weeknight meals will take even less time.

On Sunday, you can also make batches of quinoa, brown rice, and sweet potatoes to freeze. These foods take longer to prepare and are convenient to have on hand to be used throughout the meal plan. You can also purchase frozen or microwavable quinoa or brown rice if you prefer not to prepare it yourself. Sunday's leftovers (Lamb Chili) should also be frozen for use later this week and in week 3. And store your dressing for the Spinach and Strawberry Salad on the side so your leftovers don't wilt in the refrigerator. Yuck!

- ❑ Onion, white (1)
- ❑ Oranges (5)

- ❑ Shallots (2)
- ❑ Strawberries, fresh, 1 container

- ❑ Sweet potatoes (2)
- ❑ Tomatoes, cherry (1 container)

PROTEIN

- ❑ Beef, ground, ¾ pound
- ❑ Chicken breast, boneless, skinless, 1 pound
- ❑ Italian sausage, ¾ pound

- ❑ Lamb, ground, 1 pound
- ❑ Lump crabmeat, ½ pound
- ❑ Pork tenderloin, 1½ pounds

- ❑ Rotisserie chicken (1)
- ❑ Salmon, 4 (4-ounce) fillets
- ❑ Tofu, firm, 1 (14-ounce) block

OTHER

- ❑ Assorted small storage containers for veggie prep and freezer foods (optional)

Week 2

Congrats on completing week 1 and moving on to week 2! Take stock of where you are this week. Consider writing down some of the benefits you have seen. A few questions you might ask yourself include:

- Am I feeling better?
- Do I have less pain?
- Has my mobility improved?
- Have I lost weight?
- Did I find a new recipe I love?
- What were my successes last week?
- What were some of my challenges?
- What can I improve this week?

Week 2 can be when some of the motivation starts to wear off as things become routine. But this is when you will begin to see results, so it's important to stay consistent. Be kind to yourself. If you are having a particularly stressful week, focus on the easy-to-prepare or plan-ahead meals. Keep things simple!

Week 2 Meal Plan

. . . .

SUNDAY

Breakfast: Eggs Florentine Omelet with Avocado Hollandaise (page 63) and 1 slice of whole-wheat toast

Lunch: Canadian Bacon and Veggie Pita Pizzas (page 123)

Dinner: Spaghetti with Turkey Meatballs (page 107)

Snack: Maple-Glazed Baked Apples (page 140) over low-fat plain Greek yogurt

. . . .

MONDAY

Breakfast: Avocado and Egg Toasts with Pepitas (page 60) and 1½ cups of diced mango

Lunch: Leftover Spaghetti with Turkey Meatballs

Dinner: Asian Pork Tenderloin with Spicy Red Cabbage Slaw (page 118) and 1 cup of brown rice

Snack: 1 Asian pear and 2 ounces of string cheese

. . . .

TUESDAY

Breakfast: Pumpkin Pie Smoothie (page 56) and 1 slice of whole-wheat toast with 1 tablespoon of almond butter

Lunch: Leftover Asian Pork Tenderloin with Spicy Red Cabbage Slaw in 1 whole-wheat pita

Dinner: Shrimp and Broccoli Salad with Garlic Vinaigrette (page 75) over 1 cup of cooked quinoa

Snack: Trail mix: ¼ cup of dried cranberries, ¼ cup of pepitas, and ¼ cup of pecans

WEDNESDAY

Breakfast: Avocado and Egg Toasts with Pepitas (page 60) and 1 cup of grapes

Lunch: Leftover Shrimp and Broccoli Salad with Garlic Vinaigrette

Dinner: Beef and Asparagus Stir-Fry (page 128)

Snack: Leftover Maple-Glazed Baked Apples over low-fat plain Greek yogurt

THURSDAY

Breakfast: Yogurt, Berry, and Walnut Breakfast Parfait (page 58)

Lunch: Leftover Beef and Asparagus Stir-Fry and 1 cup of brown rice

Dinner: Cod and Veggies in Parchment (page 98) and 1 baked sweet potato with 1 teaspoon of butter

Snack: Trail mix: ¼ cup of dried cranberries, ¼ cup of pepitas, and ¼ cup of pecans

FRIDAY

Breakfast: Blackberry Kale Smoothie (page 55)

Lunch: Peri-Peri Shrimp and Avocado Salad (page 74) and 1 whole-wheat pita

Dinner: Leftover Cod and Veggies in Parchment and 1 baked sweet potato with 1 teaspoon of butter

Snack: Yogurt, Berry, and Walnut Breakfast Parfait (page 58)

SATURDAY

Breakfast: Open-Faced Spinach, Feta, and Tapenade Egg Sandwich (page 68)

Lunch: Leftover Peri-Peri Shrimp and Avocado Salad and 1 whole-wheat pita

Dinner: Turkey Sausage, White Bean, Kale, and Potato Soup (page 78)

Snack: Trail mix: ¼ cup of dried cranberries, ¼ cup of pepitas, and ¼ cup of pecans

WEEK 2 SHOPPING LIST

This week's shopping list builds upon last week's list. Items that should have been purchased last week, like olive oil, spices, vinegar, and bread, were not repeated. The list also assumes that you have other staples ready to go, like brown rice and quinoa.

DAIRY AND EGGS

- ❑ Cheese, string, 1 package
- ❑ Cheese, shredded mozzarella, 1 (8-ounce) bag
- ❑ Eggs, large, omega-3 fortified, 18
- ❑ Greek yogurt, low-fat, plain, 4 (5-ounce) containers
- ❑ Milk, skim (½ gallon)

CANNED AND BOTTLED ITEMS

- ❑ Artichoke hearts, 1 (14-ounce) can
- ❑ Broth, low-sodium chicken, 5 (14-ounce) cans
- ❑ Cannellini beans, 1 (14-ounce) can
- ❑ Olives, black, 2 (2.25-ounce) cans
- ❑ Olives, green, 1 small jar
- ❑ Pumpkin purée, 1 (14-ounce) can
- ❑ Tomatoes, crushed, 3 (14-ounce) cans
- ❑ Tomatoes and basil, crushed, 1 (14-ounce) can
- ❑ Vinegar, white, 1 (16-ounce) bottle

PANTRY ITEMS

- ❑ Bread, whole-wheat pita
- ❑ Chinese hot mustard
- ❑ Cinnamon, ground
- ❑ Dill, dried
- ❑ Flour
- ❑ Nutmeg, ground
- ❑ Pecans
- ❑ Pepitas (hulled pumpkin seeds)
- ❑ Peri-peri sauce

- ❏ Spaghetti (whole-wheat or gluten-free)
- ❏ Stevia
- ❏ Tarragon, dried
- ❏ Vanilla extract

PRODUCE

- ❏ Apples (4)
- ❏ Asparagus (1 bunch)
- ❏ Avocados (5)
- ❏ Baby spinach (1 bag)
- ❏ Basil, fresh (1 bunch)
- ❏ Bell peppers, red (3)
- ❏ Blueberries, fresh (1 container, or 1 bag frozen blueberries)
- ❏ Broccoli (1 head)
- ❏ Cabbage, red (1 head)
- ❏ Cilantro (1 bunch)
- ❏ Garlic (3 heads)
- ❏ Grapes (1 bunch)
- ❏ Kale, chopped (1 bag)
- ❏ Lemons (2)
- ❏ Lime (1)
- ❏ Mango (2)
- ❏ Mushrooms, shiitake (1 container)
- ❏ Onions, green (2 bunches)
- ❏ Onions, red (6)
- ❏ Parsley, Italian (1 bunch)
- ❏ Pears, Asian (3)
- ❏ Potatoes, red (4)
- ❏ Sweet potatoes (2)
- ❏ Tomatoes, cherry (1 container)
- ❏ Zucchini (1)

PROTEIN

- ❏ Beef sirloin, 1½ pounds
- ❏ Canadian bacon, 1 package
- ❏ Cod, 4 (4-ounce) fillets
- ❏ Pork tenderloin, 1½ pounds
- ❏ Shrimp, cooked, 2 pounds
- ❏ Turkey breast, ground, 1 pound
- ❏ Turkey sausage, 1 pound

OTHER

- ❏ Parchment paper

WEEK 2 TIPS

You have made it to week 2 and are hopefully learning a lot about cooking and managing your meals! This week builds upon week 1. There are several items you should have prepped and frozen from week 1 that are used this week. For example, rice, quinoa, or sweet potatoes can all be frozen and ready to go when you need. Or you can load up on precooked or microwavable starches.

A few tips to make week 2 meal prep easier:

- **Marinate the pork for Monday's dinner on Sunday.** That way it will be ready to go after a busy day.

- **You might find yourself with a little extra shrimp left over after prepping the Shrimp and Broccoli Salad with Garlic Vinaigrette and the Peri-Peri Shrimp and Avocado Salad.** Keep it frozen for the future or cook it and chill it for a shrimp cocktail snack.

- **The Turkey Sausage, White Bean, Kale, and Potato Soup leftovers will be used in week 3.** But you can make a large batch and freeze it for busy weeks ahead.

- **A few breakfast items can be used as snacks.** The smoothie recipes make two servings, so they can be split up into a breakfast and a snack. The breakfast parfait can also be a great high-protein snack later in the week, since you already have the ingredients on hand.

Week 3

Congrats! You made it to the last week of the plan. How are you feeling? Continue to look for the positives. Are your pants looser? Are you feeling less inflamed? Experiencing more mobility?

At this point you have likely lost a bit of weight and are feeling better. Even if your results are not dramatic, continue to follow the plan. It does take longer than three weeks to experience a change in symptoms, but you are on your way. The important thing is keeping up your momentum and investing in yourself. You've already proven you can do this for two weeks, so do it for two more and two more after that. Be sure you are addressing lifestyle factors, such as sleep and exercise, to see the best results.

Since this is the last week of the plan in this book, take a moment on Sunday to reflect on what has gone well and what the challenges are. Check out the "What's Next?" section (page 50) for a few ideas on how to continue to move forward with your healthier lifestyle.

Week 3 Menu

SUNDAY

Breakfast: Zucchini and Caramelized Onion Frittata (page 67) and 1 slice of whole-wheat bread with 1 teaspoon of butter

Lunch: Leftover Turkey Sausage, White Bean, Kale, and Potato Soup from week 2

Dinner: Greek-Style Pork Chops with Olive Salsa (page 122) and 1 cup of quinoa

Snack: ½ cup of black olives and 2 ounces of string cheese

MONDAY

Breakfast: Chia and Pom Breakfast Pudding (page 57)

Lunch: Leftover Zucchini and Caramelized Onion Frittata

Dinner: Leftover Greek-Style Pork Chops with Olive Salsa as a salad over lettuce and tomatoes with 2 tablespoons of olive oil dressing and 1 whole-wheat pita

Snack: 1 banana and ⅓ cup of pecans

TUESDAY

Breakfast: 1 cup of cooked oatmeal with ⅓ cup of pecans and 1 cup of mixed frozen berries

Lunch: Veggie and Hummus Pitas (page 79)

Dinner: Mushroom and Red Wine Ragout with Whole-Wheat Pasta (page 84)

Snack: Chia and Pom Breakfast Pudding (page 57)

WEDNESDAY

Breakfast: 2 slices of whole-wheat toast with 2 tablespoons of almond butter, 1 sliced banana, and pomegranate seeds

Lunch: Leftover Mushroom and Red Wine Ragout with Whole-Wheat Pasta

Dinner: Leftover Lamb Chili from week 1 with ⅓ cup of shredded cheese

Snack: 4 tablespoons of hummus with 1 cup of carrots and ½ whole-wheat pita

THURSDAY

Breakfast: Red Breakfast Hash (page 69) and 1 cup of mixed frozen berries

Lunch: Leftover Veggie and Hummus Pitas and 1 orange

Dinner: Maple and Citrus–Glazed Salmon (page 103) and 1 cup of couscous

Snack: ½ cup of black olives and 2 ounces of string cheese

FRIDAY

Breakfast: Leftover Red Breakfast Hash and 1 orange

Lunch: Rice and Bean Burritos (page 87)

Dinner: Leftover Maple and Citrus–Glazed Salmon and 1 cup of couscous

Snack: 1 banana and ⅓ cup of pecans

SATURDAY

Breakfast: Shakshuka (page 66) with 1 slice of whole-wheat toast and 1 teaspoon of butter

Lunch: Leftover Rice and Bean Burritos

Dinner: Eggplant, Bell Pepper, and Tomato Bake (page 88) and 1 baked sweet potato

Snack: 4 tablespoons of hummus with 1 cup of carrots and ½ whole-wheat pita

WEEK 3 SHOPPING LIST

Just like the shopping list for week 2, this list does not include every item featured in the recipes because they have been purchased during previous weeks. It is assumed you have items like bread, olive oil, salt, pepper, and other seasonings featured in previous recipes. Before you decide to follow this menu, take stock of what items you may have run out of.

DAIRY AND EGGS

❑ Cheese, feta, 1 (6 oz) container

❑ Cheese, shredded mozzarella or

Monterey Jack, 1 (8-ounce) package

❑ Cheese, Parmesan, 1 (8-ounce) tub

❑ Eggs, large, omega-3 fortified (2 dozen)

❑ Milk, skim or nondairy (½ gallon)

CANNED AND BOTTLED ITEMS

❑ Broth, low-sodium vegetable, 2 (14-ounce) cans

❑ Black beans, 1 (14-ounce) can

❑ Chickpeas, 2 (14-ounce) cans

❑ Olive oil–based salad dressing

❑ Olives, Spanish, 1 small jar

❑ Olives, black, 2 (2.25-ounce) cans

❑ Tahini, 1 jar

❑ Tomatoes, crushed, 3 (28-ounce) cans

PANTRY ITEMS

❑ Coriander, ground

❑ Couscous, whole grain

❑ Mushrooms, dried, 1 ounce

❑ Oatmeal

❑ Onion powder

❑ Paprika

❑ Rotini, whole-wheat

❑ Tortillas, whole-wheat, 1 package

❑ Thyme, dried

PRODUCE

- ❏ Bananas (3)
- ❏ Bell pepper, green (1)
- ❏ Bell peppers, red (3)
- ❏ Cabbage, red (1 head)
- ❏ Carrots, baby (1 bag)
- ❏ Eggplant (1)
- ❏ Garlic (2 heads)
- ❏ Kale, chopped (1 bag)
- ❏ Lemons (4)
- ❏ Lettuce (1 bag)
- ❏ Lime (1)
- ❏ Mushrooms, cremini (1 pound)
- ❏ Mushrooms, shiitake (1 pound)
- ❏ Onions, red (7)
- ❏ Oranges (4)
- ❏ Parsley or cilantro (1 bunch)
- ❏ Pomegranate (1 container shelled seeds or 1 whole pomegranate)
- ❏ Potatoes, large, red (2)
- ❏ Tomatoes, large (2)
- ❏ Tomatoes, cherry (1 container)
- ❏ Zucchini (1)

PROTEIN

- ❏ Pork, 6 boneless thin-cut chops
- ❏ Salmon, 4 (4-ounce) fillets

OTHER

- ❏ Red wine, dry, 1 bottle

WEEK 3 TIPS

At this point you should be a pro at meal prep and looking at the week ahead. As always, do as much prepping and planning as you can on Sunday. Just like you did in previous weeks, look for ways to save time by using convenience foods like pre-cut veggies, microwavable starches, or other pre-prepared items.

A few tips for the week three recipes:

- **Make the Chia and Pom Breakfast Pudding ahead of time.** It can keep in the refrigerator for up to five days. It makes a great breakfast or snack. Don't limit yourself to this exact recipe: It is quite versatile and can be topped with nuts, seeds, or a variety of fruits.

- **Make a large batch of hummus to use for meals and snacks.** Hummus can also be purchased from the store to save time.

- **When you make the Rice and Bean Burritos, consider making a double batch.** They can be frozen and used at a later time for a last-minute healthy lunch.

- **If you don't have time to make oatmeal in the morning, consider overnight oats.** Put the water or milk in the oats before you go to bed and let them sit in the refrigerator overnight.

- **This week relies on some freezer items that were prepared during week 1.** If you don't have any leftover Lamb Chili, you can pick another recipe from the book.

WHAT TO EAT WHEN YOU EAT OUT

Eating out can be a challenge for anyone. You can't control what they put in the food at restaurants, and portions are frequently way too large. But most dining establishments do offer healthy choices, if you want. Here are a few tips for eating out while following your plan:

- **Do your research.** There are many healthy options available in every city, even in quick-service restaurants. Do some local research for restaurants that offer a variety of healthier dishes.

- **Stick with meals that are made up of mostly protein and vegetables.**

- **Fish, chicken, and lean cuts of meat are great choices.**

- **Order your protein choice grilled or baked.**

- **Avoid starches like pasta and white rice when eating out.** Say no to the bread basket or chips.

- **Ask for a double side of vegetables.**

- **Watch your drinks.** Order water or unsweetened tea. Limit alcohol.

- **Consider sharing a meal or taking half home.**

- **Skip dessert.** Order fresh fruit if it's available or make a dessert from the recipe section of this book to enjoy when you get home.

- **Use eating out as inspiration.** Look for restaurants that prepare healthy fare and learn how they cook their meals.

- **If you do indulge, forgive yourself and move on.** No one can be perfect, and you shouldn't let one meal discourage you and send you back to old habits.

We all eat out sometimes. Try to make the best choice possible and focus on enjoying your meal and the experience of dining out.

What's Next?

Congratulations on completing the 21-day osteoarthritis meal plan! Now it is time to do a complete assessment of how it went and make a plan to continue to move forward. Start by asking yourself a few check-in questions:

- What went well during the last three weeks?
- What was challenging?
- Do you feel better overall?
- Do you have less joint pain?
- Do you have less joint stiffness?
- Has your energy improved?
- Are you sleeping better?
- If you needed to, have you lost weight?
- Which meals were easy to prepare on this meal plan?
- Which meals were difficult?
- Which meals were tastiest to you?
- Which meals would you make again?

Once you have a deep understanding of how things went and where you are right now, you can start to create a plan to help you move forward. There are many other recipes in the book that you may not have tried yet. These can be a starting point for you to create your own weekly meal plans.

The secret to maintaining a healthy diet and lifestyle is twofold: awareness and planning. First, you need to become aware of the less-than-ideal choices you are making. Many of us eat mindlessly. We don't give much thought to what we are putting in our mouths on a regular basis. We do little planning and tend to end up in situations where unhealthy food is the only (or easiest) option. We don't prioritize our days to focus on what's truly important.

Everyone has busy weeks, everyone has responsibilities they need to deal with, and everyone is crunched for time. It is easy to get wrapped up in other areas of life. But can you really give 100 percent to these other areas if you are not healthy? If you are in constant pain? Health needs to be a priority because when health fails, everything else fails, too.

You can start making positive changes, but first you have to be aware of your challenges. Awareness allows you to start coming up with better solutions. When you really take a look at the lifestyle choices that are not serving you and create a plan to change those habits, you'll see success.

Health is not just about what you eat. All aspects of your lifestyle, such as stress, sleep, and exercise, also need to be addressed for true health. Diet can be one step in the right direction toward reducing pain and living a better life. But don't stop there. Continue to look at other ways you can focus on health and the journey toward the life you truly want.

Shakshuka, page 66

CHAPTER 4

Breakfast & Smoothies

Blueberry, Spinach, and Almond Butter Smoothie

QUICK & EASY SERVES 2 / PREP TIME: 5 MINUTES

Smoothies are a great way to get your day started right. With the antioxidants in blueberries and spinach and the fatty almond butter to fill you up, this smoothie will satisfy you and carry you through your morning with energy and ease. Split the smoothie with a loved one or refrigerate the rest for a snack or tomorrow's breakfast.

2 cups nonfat milk or unsweetened nondairy milk such as almond milk

2 teaspoons matcha powder (optional)

2 tablespoons almond butter

2 cups frozen blueberries

2 cups baby spinach

In a blender, combine all ingredients. Cover and blend until smooth, 30 seconds to 1 minute.

THE GOOD STUFF: Blueberries are filled with anthocyanins, which have been shown to reduce pain associated with arthritis, while the optional matcha is a good energy booster that also contains EGCG. You can find matcha powder in the tea aisle of most grocery stores, online, or in health food stores.

PER SERVING: Calories: 270; Total fat: 10g; Saturated fat: 1g; Carbohydrates: 36g; Fiber: 7g; Protein: 12g

Blackberry Kale Smoothie

QUICK & EASY **SERVES 2 / PREP TIME: 5 MINUTES**

Frozen blackberries thicken up this tasty smoothie, while chia seeds add beneficial omega-3 fatty acids. As with the previous smoothie, matcha powder is added as an optional ingredient, both as an energy boost and for the EGCG it contains. If this smoothie is too thick, add a little water to thin it to your liking.

2 cups nonfat milk or unsweetened nondairy milk

2 tablespoons chia seeds

2 teaspoons matcha powder (optional)

2 cups frozen blackberries

1 cup chopped kale, stems removed

1. In a blender, combine the milk and chia seeds. Allow to sit for 5 minutes.
2. Add the matcha powder (if using), blackberries, and kale. Cover and blend until smooth.

SUBSTITUTION TIP: Don't have matcha powder? Brew a strong cup of green tea and chill it overnight. Then reduce the milk by ½ cup and add the tea instead.

PER SERVING: Calories: 258; Total fat: 4g; Saturated fat: <1g; Carbohydrates: 45g; Fiber: 14g; Protein: 14g

Pumpkin Pie Smoothie

QUICK & EASY **SERVES 2 / PREP TIME: 5 MINUTES**

If you're a fan of the pumpkin spice trend, then this is the healthy breakfast smoothie for you. With the fall flavors of pumpkin, cinnamon, ginger, and vanilla, it's a delicious start to your day that tastes a little like dessert. It also sneaks in plenty of fiber.

2 cups nonfat milk or unsweetened nondairy milk

¼ cup pepitas

1 cup canned pumpkin purée (not pumpkin pie filling)

2 packets of stevia or 2 tablespoons pure maple syrup

½ teaspoon pure vanilla extract

½ teaspoon freshly grated ginger

½ teaspoon ground cinnamon

½ cup ice

In a blender, combine all ingredients. Blend until smooth.

THE GOOD STUFF: Ginger has a whole host of health benefits, including some reported potential help for people with osteoarthritis. If you don't have fresh ginger, ground ginger will work as well. Pepitas (hulled pumpkin seeds) are a decent source of omega-3 fatty acids.

PER SERVING: Calories: 218; Total fat: 8g; Saturated fat: 1g; Carbohydrates: 23g; Fiber: 6g; Protein: 16g

Chia and Pom Breakfast Pudding

QUICK & EASY, MAKE AHEAD SERVES 2 / PREP TIME: 5 MINUTES, PLUS 8 HOURS TO REST

Chia seeds expand in liquid to make a pudding that is similar in texture to tapioca. This breakfast pudding is lightly sweet, and the chia helps carry you through the morning. Make it the night before, and it will be ready for you in the morning. It will keep in the refrigerator for up to four days.

2 cups nonfat milk or unsweetened nondairy milk

2 tablespoons pure maple syrup or 2 packets of stevia

½ teaspoon ground cinnamon

½ teaspoon pure vanilla extract

2 tablespoons chia seeds

1 cup pomegranate arils (seeds)

1. In a mason jar, combine the milk, syrup, cinnamon, and vanilla. Cover and shake to mix.
2. Add the chia seeds and stir. Cover and refrigerate overnight. The chia seeds will expand, and it will thicken into pudding.
3. In the morning, sprinkle ½ cup pomegranate seeds over each serving.

COOKING TIP: You can buy pomegranate arils already removed from the fruit in the refrigerated part of the produce section, or you can remove them from the pomegranate yourself. To do so, halve the pomegranate and hold it with the cut section over a bowl. Tap firmly on the uncut part of the pomegranate with a wooden spoon to release the arils.

PER SERVING: Calories: 272; Total fat: 4g; Saturated fat: <1g; Carbohydrates: 47g; Fiber: 8g; Protein: 12g

Yogurt, Berry, and Walnut Breakfast Parfait

QUICK & EASY, MAKE AHEAD **SERVES 1 / PREP TIME: 5 MINUTES**

Greek yogurt is a protein powerhouse that fills you up and keeps you going throughout the morning. This simple breakfast parfait gets its sweetness from berries, but you can add a teaspoon of honey or pure maple syrup to the yogurt to sweeten it up a bit if you have a sweet tooth.

¾ cup Greek yogurt

1 cup fresh blueberries

¼ cup walnut pieces

1 tablespoon honey or pure maple syrup (optional)

1. In a parfait glass or bowl, layer half the yogurt on the bottom.
2. Add half the blueberries and half the walnut pieces.
3. Add another layer with the remaining yogurt.
4. Add the remaining blueberries and walnut pieces.
5. Drizzle with honey or pure maple syrup, if desired.

SUBSTITUTION TIP: Raspberries, strawberries, blackberries, pomegranate seeds, or any other sliced fruit will also work with this recipe if you want to mix it up a little. You can even use mixed berries, such as ½ cup of blueberries and ½ cup of raspberries.

PER SERVING: Calories: 456; Total fat: 29g; Saturated fat: 6g; Carbohydrates: 32g; Fiber: 6g; Protein: 22g

Overnight Oats with Dried Cranberries

QUICK & EASY, MAKE AHEAD **SERVES 2 / PREP TIME: 5 MINUTES, PLUS 8 HOURS TO REST**

Overnight oats are an easy, creamy breakfast option. They require almost no prep time, and there's very little cleanup since no equipment other than a covered bowl is required. Don't feel limited by this recipe: Once you get the hang of overnight oats, you can experiment with adding your favorite fruits or nuts.

½ cup rolled oats

½ cup nonfat milk or unsweetened nondairy milk

1 tablespoon chia seeds

¼ cup Greek yogurt

2 tablespoons pure maple syrup or 2 packets of stevia

½ cup dried cranberries

1. In a small bowl, combine the oats, milk, chia seeds, yogurt, and maple syrup.
2. Stir, cover, and refrigerate overnight.
3. Stir in the cranberries just before serving.

SUBSTITUTION TIP: Try using dried cherries or dried blueberries. Fresh fruit works well here, too. Add up to 1 cup of sliced strawberries, blueberries, blackberries, or raspberries.

PER SERVING: Calories: 306; Total fat: 5g; Saturated fat: 1g; Carbohydrates: 58g; Fiber: 5g; Protein: 9g

Avocado and Egg Toasts with Pepitas

QUICK & EASY **SERVES 4 / PREP TIME: 5 MINUTES / COOK TIME: 5 MINUTES**

This is a quick and easy breakfast. It works for a weekday, or you might want to enjoy it on a leisurely weekend morning while curled up with the weekend paper. While this recipe calls for you to cook the eggs over easy, you can cook them any way you like.

1 tablespoon extra-virgin olive oil

4 large eggs

Sea salt

Freshly cracked black pepper

4 tablespoons pepitas (hulled pumpkin seeds)

1 avocado, peeled, pitted, and mashed

4 slices whole-wheat bread, toasted

1. In a nonstick cooking pan, heat the olive oil on medium-low until it shimmers. Reduce the heat to low and gently crack the eggs into the pan.
2. Season lightly with salt and pepper.
3. Without moving the eggs, allow the whites to set on the heat, about 3 minutes.
4. Turn off the heat and carefully flip the eggs. Allow to sit in contact with the pan for 30 seconds for over easy, or about 1 minute for over-medium.
5. Meanwhile, stir the pepitas into the mashed avocado and spread it on the toast.
6. Top with the eggs.

SUBSTITUTION TIP: If you like your food on the spicy side, add a dash of cayenne to the avocados or dash your favorite hot sauce on top of the eggs. If you need to be gluten-free, substitute with gluten-free bread for the toast.

PER SERVING: Calories: 309; Total fat: 20g; Saturated fat: 4g; Carbohydrates: 23g; Fiber: 3g; Protein: 14g

Make-Ahead Egg, Red Onion, and Brussels Sprout Breakfast "Muffins"

MAKE AHEAD, LEFTOVERS LUNCH

MAKES 6 MUFFINS / PREP TIME: 10 MINUTES / COOK TIME: 20 MINUTES

. . . .

These breakfast "muffins" freeze well, so if you have a larger muffin tin, you can double the batch, freeze them in zip-top bags, and thaw one and reheat it in the microwave for breakfast or for a snack. They'll also keep in the refrigerator for about four days, so it's a great way to have a hot breakfast even on weekdays. Two muffins make one serving.

. . . .

Nonstick cooking spray

2 tablespoons extra-virgin olive oil

½ red onion, finely chopped

2 cups chopped Brussels sprouts

6 large eggs

¼ teaspoon garlic powder

½ teaspoon Dijon mustard

½ teaspoon sea salt

⅛ teaspoon freshly cracked black pepper

Dash Tabasco or your favorite hot sauce (optional)

1. Preheat your oven to 375°F. Spray a 6-cup muffin tin with nonstick cooking spray or line it with silicone tin liners.
2. In a medium nonstick skillet, heat the olive oil on medium-high until it shimmers.
3. Add the red onion and Brussels sprouts. Cook, stirring occasionally, until the vegetables soften, about 5 minutes. Remove from heat and allow to cool.
4. In a bowl, beat the eggs with the garlic powder, mustard, salt, pepper, and Tabasco (if using).
5. Stir in the cooled vegetables.
6. Distribute the mixture evenly in the prepared muffin tins. Bake until the eggs set, about 18 minutes.

. . . .

SUBSTITUTION TIP: If you don't fancy Brussels sprouts, you can also use 2 cups of shredded red cabbage or even shredded coleslaw mix (minus the dressing).

. . . .

PER SERVING (2 MUFFINS): Calories: 258; Total fat: 19g; Saturated fat: 5g; Carbohydrates: 8g; Fiber: 3g; Protein: 15g

Quick Broccoli, Kale, and Egg Scramble

QUICK & EASY, ONE POT SERVES 2 / PREP TIME: 10 MINUTES / COOK TIME: 10 MINUTES

It doesn't take long to scramble eggs and veggies, making this a good breakfast on the go or for a more leisurely weekend meal. This breakfast also feels hearty even though it's light and full of fiber. If you're cooking for one, refrigerate leftovers overnight to reheat for tomorrow's breakfast in the microwave.

2 tablespoons extra-virgin olive oil

½ red onion, finely chopped

1 cup broccoli florets

1 cup chopped kale, stems removed

½ red bell pepper, seeds and ribs removed, finely chopped

4 large eggs

¼ teaspoon sea salt

⅛ teaspoon freshly cracked black pepper

1. In a large, nonstick skillet, heat the olive oil on medium-high until it shimmers.
2. Add the onion, broccoli, kale, and red bell pepper. Cook, stirring occasionally, until the vegetables soften, about 5 minutes.
3. In a small bowl, beat the eggs with the salt and pepper.
4. Reduce the heat in the pan to medium and pour in the eggs. Cook, stirring, until the eggs set, about 3 minutes more.

THE GOOD STUFF: Red bell peppers and red onions are rich in anthocyanins while the broccoli and kale are rich in both quercetin and sulforaphane, all of which have shown promise in easing the symptoms of osteoarthritis.

PER SERVING: Calories: 315; Total fat: 24g; Saturated fat: 5g; Carbohydrates: 11g; Fiber: 3g; Protein: 15g

Eggs Florentine Omelet with Avocado Hollandaise

SERVES 4 / PREP TIME: 15 MINUTES / COOK TIME: 10 MINUTES

. . . .

While traditional eggs Florentine are made with poached egg, this omelet makes the process quick, easy, and foolproof. You'll get all the tasty flavor of eggs Florentine, but it's lower in fat and calories than the typical recipe. An avocado hollandaise is much easier than a traditional hollandaise, since it isn't at risk of breaking.

. . . .

FOR THE OMELET

2 tablespoons extra-virgin olive oil, divided

½ red onion, minced

½ red bell pepper, seeds and ribs removed, finely chopped

3 cups baby spinach

½ teaspoon sea salt, divided

Pinch freshly grated nutmeg

2 garlic cloves, minced

6 large eggs

⅛ teaspoon freshly cracked black pepper

TO MAKE THE OMELET

1. In a nonstick skillet, heat 1 tablespoon of olive oil on medium-high until it shimmers.
2. Add the onion and bell pepper and cook, stirring, until the vegetables are soft, about 5 minutes.
3. Add the spinach, half the salt, the nutmeg, and the garlic. Cook until the spinach softens, just 1 to 2 minutes.
4. Spoon the veggies into a bowl and use a paper towel to wipe out the pan.
5. Return it to medium-high heat and add the remaining 1 tablespoon of olive oil. Heat until the oil shimmers.
6. In a bowl, whisk the eggs with the remaining salt and the pepper.
7. Pour into the pan.
8. Allow to cook without stirring on medium-high until the eggs set around the edges. Use a spatula to carefully pull the edges away from the sides of the pan and tilt the pan to allow uncooked egg to flow into the gaps.
9. Cook until the edges set again. Spoon the spinach mixture over the top and flip the omelet. Cook briefly (1 minute or so) to allow the filling to reheat.

CONTINUED ▸

FOR THE HOLLANDAISE

⅓ cup boiling water

½ avocado, peeled, pitted, and chopped

2 teaspoons freshly squeezed lemon juice

Sea salt

Freshly cracked black pepper

2 tablespoons extra-virgin olive oil

TO MAKE THE HOLLANDAISE

1. In a blender, combine the boiling water, avocado, lemon juice, and salt and pepper to taste. Blend until smooth.
2. With the blender still running, pour the olive oil slowly into the mixture in a thin stream until all the olive oil is incorporated.
3. Spoon over the omelet.

SUBSTITUTION TIP: Don't feel like making your own hollandaise? You can also use 2 tablespoons of prepared guacamole on top of the omelet in its place.

PER SERVING: Calories: 283; Total fat: 25g; Saturated fat: 5g; Carbohydrates: 6g; Fiber: 3g; Protein: 11g

Mediterranean Breakfast Tostada

SERVES 4 / PREP TIME: 15 MINUTES / COOK TIME: 20 MINUTES

White bean purée serves as a tasty substitute for refried beans in this fresh and flavorful breakfast tostada with Mediterranean flavors and a hint of spice. If you like breakfast burritos, this is a delicious and fresh take on them. It calls for corn tortillas, so this recipe is gluten-free.

FOR THE PURÉE

1 (14-ounce) can low-sodium cannellini beans (white kidney beans), drained

3 garlic cloves, minced

Juice of 1 lemon, freshly squeezed

Pinch cayenne pepper

2 tablespoons extra-virgin olive oil

¼ teaspoon sea salt

FOR THE TOSTADA

4 soft corn tortillas

1 tablespoon extra-virgin olive oil

½ red onion, finely minced

1 cup sliced mushrooms

½ red bell pepper, seeds and ribs removed, finely chopped

2 garlic cloves, minced

½ teaspoon sea salt

6 large eggs, beaten

1 cup cherry tomatoes, halved

½ cup feta cheese crumbles

TO MAKE THE PURÉE

1. In a blender or food processor, combine all ingredients.
2. Blend until smooth.

TO MAKE THE TOSTADA

1. Preheat your oven to 275°F. Wrap the corn tortillas in foil and place them in the oven to warm for 20 minutes.
2. Meanwhile, in a nonstick skillet, heat the olive oil on medium-high until it shimmers.
3. Add the red onion, mushrooms, and bell pepper. Cook, stirring occasionally, until the vegetables are soft, about 5 minutes.
4. Add the garlic and the salt and cook, stirring, for 30 seconds.
5. Add the eggs and cook, stirring, until the eggs set, 2 to 3 minutes.
6. Spread the bean purée on the warmed corn tortillas. Top with the eggs.
7. Sprinkle with tomatoes and feta.

SUBSTITUTION TIP: You can substitute whole-wheat toast or gluten-free toast for the tortillas if you prefer to have an open-faced sandwich instead.

PER SERVING: Calories: 412; Total fat: 23g; Saturated fat: 7g; Carbohydrates: 36g; Fiber: 8g; Protein: 21g

Shakshuka

ONE POT **SERVES 4 / PREP TIME: 15 MINUTES / COOK TIME: 15 MINUTES**

Shakshuka is a healthy, fiber-rich egg dish in which eggs are poached in a spicy tomato sauce. Feel free to substitute spices or make it spicier or less spicy depending on your personal tastes. This easy one-pot recipe is sure to become a family favorite.

2 tablespoons extra-virgin olive oil

1 red onion, diced

1 red bell pepper, seeds and ribs removed, diced

4 garlic cloves, minced

¼ teaspoon chili powder

¼ teaspoon ground coriander

2 teaspoons paprika (or smoked paprika)

1 teaspoon ground cumin

Pinch cayenne pepper

1 (28-ounce) can crushed tomatoes, undrained

½ teaspoon sea salt

⅛ teaspoon freshly cracked black pepper

4 large eggs

¼ cup chopped fresh parsley or cilantro

1. In a large, nonstick pan, heat the olive oil on medium-high until it shimmers.
2. Add the onions and bell pepper. Cook, stirring occasionally, until the vegetables soften, about 4 minutes.
3. Add the garlic and cook, stirring constantly, for 1 minute.
4. Add the chili powder, coriander, paprika, cumin, and cayenne. Cook, stirring, for 1 minute.
5. Add the tomatoes, salt, and pepper. Bring to a simmer, stirring.
6. Using a spoon, make 4 wells in the tomato sauce. Carefully crack an egg into each well and spoon the sauce around the edges of the eggs with most of the white and yolk still showing.
7. Cover and cook until the eggs set, 5 to 9 minutes.
8. Sprinkle with the freshly chopped herbs.

SUBSTITUTION TIP: This is also very good with fresh crumbled feta on it. Sprinkle a few tablespoons of feta over the top just before you serve.

PER SERVING: Calories: 231; Total fat: 12g; Saturated fat: 3g; Carbohydrates: 21g; Fiber: 5g; Protein: 11g

Zucchini and Caramelized Onion Frittata

ONE POT SERVES 4 / PREP TIME: 15 MINUTES / COOK TIME: 20 MINUTES

Caramelized onions add deep, rich flavors to this frittata, a popular Italian egg dish. You'll need an ovenproof skillet to prepare this, since you move it from the stovetop to the oven for the final step. To make the onions caramelize quickly, slice them as thinly as you can.

2 tablespoons extra-virgin olive oil

1 red onion, thinly sliced

1 zucchini, chopped

½ teaspoon dried thyme

½ teaspoon sea salt

⅛ teaspoon freshly cracked black pepper

8 large eggs

½ teaspoon Dijon mustard

¼ cup crumbled feta cheese

1. Preheat your oven's broiler on high.
2. In a large, ovenproof skillet, heat the olive oil on medium-high until it shimmers.
3. Reduce the heat to medium-low. Add the onion. Cook, stirring occasionally, until the onion is deeply browned and caramelized, about 10 minutes.
4. Add the zucchini, thyme, salt, and pepper and cook, stirring, until it softens, about 3 minutes more.
5. Meanwhile, in a bowl, whisk the eggs with the Dijon mustard.
6. Turn the pan up to medium. Arrange the vegetables neatly in the bottom of the skillet.
7. Pour in the eggs. Cook without stirring until the edges of the eggs set.
8. Use a spatula to gently pull the set eggs away from the edges of the pan. Tilt the pan to allow the uncooked eggs to flow into the spaces you made along the edges.
9. Allow the edges to set again. Sprinkle with the feta.
10. Transfer the pan to under the broiler. Cook until the eggs puff and the cheese melts slightly, about 2 minutes.
11. Slice into wedges to serve.

SUBSTITUTION TIP: If zucchini isn't in season, you can substitute 1 cup of any type of chopped winter squash, eggplant, or sweet potato.

PER SERVING: Calories: 248; Total fat: 19g; Saturated fat: 6g; Carbohydrates: 5g; Fiber: 1g; Protein: 15g

Open-Faced Spinach, Feta, and Tapenade Egg Sandwich

SERVES 4 / PREP TIME: 15 MINUTES / COOK TIME: 10 MINUTES

You can make your own simple tapenade as indicated below, or you can purchase premade tapenade at the grocery store. Making your own allows you to control the types of fats you use and how much salt it contains. If you have a few extra minutes, making your own is a healthier option.

FOR THE TAPENADE

1 cup black or green olives, pitted and finely chopped

¼ cup finely chopped fresh Italian parsley

2 tablespoons extra-virgin olive oil

1 garlic clove, minced

¼ teaspoon red pepper flakes

FOR THE SANDWICHES

4 slices whole-wheat bread, toasted

2 tablespoons extra-virgin olive oil

½ red onion, finely chopped

2 cups baby spinach

8 large eggs, beaten

½ teaspoon sea salt

⅛ teaspoon black pepper

½ cup crumbled feta cheese

TO MAKE THE TAPENADE

Combine all ingredients in a blender or food processor. Pulse for 20 one-second pulses to chop and blend.

TO MAKE THE SANDWICHES

1. Spread the tapenade on the toast.
2. In a large, nonstick skillet, heat the olive oil on medium-high until it shimmers.
3. Add the onion. Cook, stirring occasionally, until it softens, about 3 minutes.
4. Add the spinach and cook until it is soft, about 2 minutes more.
5. Add the eggs, salt, and pepper. Cook, stirring, until the eggs set, about 4 minutes.
6. Spoon over the tapenade on the toast. Top with the crumbled feta cheese.

SUBSTITUTION TIP: If you need to be gluten-free, substitute gluten-free bread or bagels for the whole-wheat bread.

PER SERVING: Calories: 452; Total fat: 32g; Saturated fat: 8g; Carbohydrates: 22g; Fiber: 4g; Protein: 20g

Red Breakfast Hash

QUICK & EASY **SERVES 4 / PREP TIME: 15 MINUTES / COOK TIME: 30 MINUTES**

Bring a little color to your morning (and get a good dose of anthocyanins) with this red breakfast hash. The potatoes take a little while to cook, so this is the perfect weekend breakfast when you top it with a quickly fried egg. Grating the potatoes with the skin on makes them cook more quickly.

3 tablespoons extra-virgin olive oil, divided

2 large red potatoes, skin on, grated

1 red onion, thinly sliced

2 cups shredded red cabbage

½ teaspoon sea salt, plus more for seasoning

⅛ teaspoon freshly cracked black pepper

2 garlic cloves, minced

4 large eggs

1. In a large, nonstick skillet, heat 2 tablespoons of olive oil on medium-high until it shimmers.
2. Reduce the heat to medium. Add the potatoes, onion, cabbage, ½ teaspoon salt, pepper, and garlic. Cook, stirring occasionally, until the vegetables brown, 15 to 20 minutes.
3. In another nonstick pan, heat the remaining tablespoon of olive oil on medium-low until it shimmers. Reduce the temperature to low.
4. Crack the eggs carefully into the pan. Season with a pinch of salt. Cook without touching them until the whites set, 3 to 4 minutes.
5. Turn off the heat under the pan. Carefully flip the eggs. Allow the eggs to sit in contact with the pan for about 30 seconds for over easy or 1 minute for over medium.
6. Serve the hash with the eggs placed on top.

THE GOOD STUFF: Red onions do double duty with osteoarthritis, adding diallyl disulfide and quercetin, both of which have been shown to positively impact osteoarthritis.

PER SERVING: Calories: 313; Total fat: 16g; Saturated fat: 3g; Carbohydrates: 35g; Fiber: 6g; Protein: 10g

Peri-Peri Shrimp and Avocado Salad, page 74

CHAPTER 5

Salads, Soups & Sandwiches

Spinach and Strawberry Salad

QUICK & EASY **SERVES 4 / PREP TIME: 10 MINUTES**

Spinach and strawberry may sound like an odd combination, but with a balsamic chia dressing, walnuts, and a bit of feta, this sweet, sour, and savory salad hits all the right notes. Chia seeds are also full of omega-3 fatty acids. If you make the salad ahead, don't add the dressing until just before you serve it.

4 cups baby spinach

1 cup sliced strawberries

½ red onion, thinly sliced

½ cup chopped walnuts

½ cup crumbled feta cheese

3 tablespoons extra-virgin olive oil

¼ cup balsamic vinegar

1 tablespoon pure maple syrup or honey

1 tablespoon chia seeds

½ teaspoon sea salt

⅛ teaspoon freshly cracked black pepper

1. In a large bowl, combine the spinach, strawberries, onion, walnuts, and feta.
2. In a small bowl, whisk together the olive oil, vinegar, syrup, chia, salt, and pepper.
3. Toss the dressing with the salad.

SUBSTITUTION TIP: If you don't have balsamic vinegar, you can substitute red wine vinegar or apple cider vinegar.

PER SERVING: Calories: 301; Total fat: 25g; Saturated fat: 5g; Carbohydrates: 15g; Fiber: 5g; Protein: 7g

Red Cabbage, Ginger, and Apple Asian Slaw

QUICK & EASY **SERVES 4 / PREP TIME: 10 MINUTES**

This slaw is delicious as a light meal by itself or served with steamed fish or baked chicken. The combination of red cabbage, apples, and ginger is a classically delicious pairing that is loaded with flavor. If you make it ahead, don't mix the dressing with the slaw until just before you eat it.

4 cups shredded red cabbage

1 apple, peeled, cored, and julienned

½ red onion, thinly sliced

¼ cup chopped fresh cilantro

3 tablespoons extra-virgin olive oil

¼ cup apple cider vinegar

2 tablespoons freshly grated ginger

3 garlic cloves, finely minced

Dash sriracha, hot sauce, cayenne pepper, or red pepper flakes

½ teaspoon sea salt

1. In a large bowl, mix the cabbage, apple, onion, and cilantro.
2. In a small bowl, whisk together the olive oil, vinegar, ginger, garlic, hot sauce to taste, and salt.
3. Toss the dressing with the salad.

COOKING TIP: Grate the red cabbage on a box grater or run it through a grating blade in a food processor to create small, even pieces of cabbage.

PER SERVING: Calories: 142; Total fat: 11g; Saturated fat: 2g; Carbohydrates: 13g; Fiber: 3g; Protein: 2g

Peri-Peri Shrimp and Avocado Salad

QUICK & EASY **SERVES 4 / PREP TIME: 10 MINUTES**

Peri-peri sauce is a southern African sauce made of peppers, garlic, and some type of acid like lemon or vinegar. You can buy it online or in the condiment section of the grocery store. It's delicious on seafood, chicken, or eggs, and it adds a little bit of spice to this flavorful shrimp salad.

1 pound cooked bay shrimp

1 avocado, peeled, pitted, and cubed

1 mango, peeled, pitted, and cubed

½ red onion, finely chopped

Juice of ½ lime

2 tablespoons prepared peri-peri sauce (see headnote)

3 tablespoons olive oil mayonnaise or Greek yogurt

¼ cup chopped fresh cilantro

1. In a large bowl, mix the shrimp, avocado, mango, and red onion. Drizzle with the lime juice and mix well.
2. In a small bowl, whisk together the peri-peri sauce and mayonnaise. Mix with the salad.
3. Top with the chopped fresh cilantro.

SUBSTITUTION TIP: Reduce fat and calories by replacing the mayonnaise with an equal amount of Greek yogurt. If you can't find peri-peri sauce, substitute your favorite hot sauce instead.

PER SERVING: Calories: 322; Total fat: 19g; Saturated fat: 3g; Carbohydrates: 15g; Fiber: 4g; Protein: 25g

Shrimp and Broccoli Salad with Garlic Vinaigrette

QUICK & EASY **SERVES 4 / PREP TIME: 10 MINUTES**

This salad makes a delicious no-cook meal. It's quick and easy to prepare, particularly if you buy your broccoli already cut into florets in the prepped veggie section of the grocery store. Unlike other salads, this one sits with the dressing on it for about 30 minutes so the broccoli can absorb the flavor.

12 ounces cooked bay shrimp

4 cups broccoli florets

½ red onion, thinly sliced

2 cups cherry tomatoes, halved

¼ cup extra-virgin olive oil

½ cup apple cider vinegar

6 garlic cloves, finely minced

1 tablespoon Dijon mustard

1 teaspoon dried tarragon

½ teaspoon sea salt

⅛ teaspoon freshly cracked black pepper

Pinch red pepper flakes

1. In a large bowl, mix the shrimp, broccoli, onion, and tomatoes.
2. In a small bowl, whisk together the olive oil, vinegar, garlic, mustard, tarragon, salt, black pepper, and red pepper flakes.
3. Toss the dressing with the salad and let sit 30 minutes in the refrigerator before serving.

COOKING TIP: You can buy premade bagged broccoli slaw and replace the broccoli florets to save time and make the broccoli have smaller bites in the salad. You'll find broccoli slaw in the prebagged salad section at the grocery store.

PER SERVING: Calories: 266; Total fat: 15g; Saturated fat: 2g; Carbohydrates: 10g; Fiber: 3g; Protein: 20g

Chopped Chicken Salad

QUICK & EASY **SERVES 4 / PREP TIME: 10 MINUTES**

Using rotisserie chicken from the grocery store makes this salad quick and easy. Remove the skin and bones and chop the chicken meat. Save what you don't use in a zip-top bag in the freezer to use by itself or to use in other recipes from this book.

2 cups chopped chicken meat

1 (14-ounce) can low-sodium kidney beans, drained

½ red onion, finely chopped

1 (14-ounce) can artichoke hearts, drained and chopped

½ cup black olives, pitted and chopped

1 red bell pepper, seeds and ribs removed, chopped

3 tablespoons extra-virgin olive oil

1 tablespoon Dijon mustard

3 garlic cloves, minced

½ cup red wine vinegar

½ teaspoon sea salt

⅛ teaspoon freshly cracked black pepper

1. In a large bowl, combine the chicken, kidney beans, onion, artichoke hearts, olives, and bell pepper.
2. In a small bowl, whisk together the olive oil, mustard, garlic, vinegar, salt, and pepper. Pour over the vegetables and chicken and toss.

THE GOOD STUFF: The olives and the olive oil used in the dressing mean this salad is loaded with beneficial oleocanthal, which can help lessen the pain of osteoarthritis.

PER SERVING: Calories: 384; Total fat: 18g; Saturated fat: 3g; Carbohydrates: 27g; Fiber: 9g; Protein: 28g

Cream of Asparagus Soup

QUICK & EASY, ONE POT **SERVES 4 / PREP TIME: 5 MINUTES / COOK TIME: 15 MINUTES**

Cream of asparagus is a light vegetarian soup with lots of flavor. You can even make this recipe vegan by replacing the yogurt with any unflavored nondairy milk. If you can find fresh dill, it has much better flavor than dried dill: Add it at the end after the soup has cooked instead of during the cooking process.

2 tablespoons extra-virgin olive oil

1 shallot, finely minced (or ½ red onion, finely chopped)

2 pounds asparagus, woody bottoms removed, chopped

3 garlic cloves, minced

3 cups low-sodium vegetable broth

1 teaspoon dried dill

½ teaspoon sea salt

⅛ teaspoon freshly cracked black pepper

½ cup Greek yogurt

1. In a large pot, heat the olive oil on medium-high until it shimmers.
2. Add the shallot and asparagus and cook, stirring occasionally, until the asparagus starts to soften, about 5 minutes.
3. Add the garlic and cook, stirring constantly, for 30 seconds.
4. Add the vegetable broth, dill, salt, and pepper. Bring to a simmer and reduce the heat to medium-low. Simmer, stirring occasionally, for 10 minutes.
5. Transfer into a blender and purée (see tip below). Add the Greek yogurt and purée again.

COOKING TIP: To purée in a blender, fold a towel and place it over the blender top. Place your hand on top of the towel and turn on the blender. Blend for about 30 seconds and then open the lid away from your face to allow the steam to escape. Put the lid on the blender, use the towel, and blend again. Do this two or three times until the soup is puréed. You need to let the steam escape, so you don't wind up with hot soup building up pressure and blowing the lid off the blender.

PER SERVING: Calories: 161; Total fat: 9g; Saturated fat: 2g; Carbohydrates: 16g; Fiber: 6g; Protein: 8g

Turkey Sausage, White Bean, Kale, and Potato Soup

ONE POT, MAKE AHEAD **SERVES 6 / PREP TIME: 15 MINUTES / COOK TIME: 20 MINUTES**

This delicious and hearty soup is easy to make ahead, and it gets even tastier when it sits in the refrigerator overnight. It freezes well—just freeze it in single servings and reheat in the microwave or on the stovetop. It's packed with flavor and is good as a lunch or dinner.

2 tablespoons extra-virgin olive oil

1 pound bulk turkey Italian sausage

1 red onion, finely chopped

4 garlic cloves, minced

3 tablespoons flour

8 cups low-sodium chicken broth

4 red potatoes, chopped

2 cups kale, stems removed, chopped

1 (14-ounce) can low-sodium cannellini beans, drained

1 teaspoon dried Italian herbs

½ teaspoon sea salt

¼ teaspoon freshly cracked black pepper

Pinch red pepper flakes

½ cup skim milk

1. In a large pot, heat the olive oil on medium-high until it shimmers.
2. Add the sausage and cook, stirring and crumbling, until it's browned, about 5 minutes.
3. Add the onion and cook, stirring, until it softens, about 3 minutes.
4. Add the garlic and cook, stirring constantly, for 30 seconds.
5. Add the flour and cook, stirring constantly, for 1 minute.
6. Add the chicken broth. Stirring constantly, bring to a simmer.
7. Reduce the heat to medium. Stir in the potatoes, kale, beans, herbs, salt, black pepper, and red pepper flakes. Simmer, stirring occasionally, until the potatoes soften, about 10 minutes.
8. Stir in the milk just before serving.

COOKING TIP: For a thinner, brothier soup, or if you need the soup to be gluten-free, omit the flour and leave out the skim milk.

PER SERVING: Calories: 363; Total fat: 12g; Saturated fat: 2g; Carbohydrates: 44g; Fiber: 8g; Protein: 23g

Veggie and Hummus Pitas

QUICK & EASY SERVES 2 / PREP TIME: 15 MINUTES

. . . .

You can substitute premade hummus for the homemade if you want to save time or ingredients. Hummus is easy to make, but since not many other things use tahini, it may not be worth it to you to buy a jar of tahini unless you plan to make a ton of hummus.

. . . .

FOR THE HUMMUS

1 (14-ounce) can low-sodium chickpeas, drained

2 garlic cloves, minced

2 tablespoons tahini

Juice of 1 lemon

½ teaspoon sea salt

¼ cup extra-virgin olive oil

FOR THE PITAS

8 tablespoons hummus (above)

2 pitas, halved

½ cup kale, stems removed, chopped

4 thin slices red onion

8 cherry tomatoes, halved

4 slices red bell pepper

TO MAKE THE HUMMUS

In a blender or food processor, combine all ingredients and blend until smooth.

TO MAKE THE PITAS

1. Spread 2 tablespoons of hummus on the inside of each pita.
2. Add the kale, onion, tomatoes, and bell pepper.

. . . .

COOKING TIP: You can save any leftover hummus in the refrigerator for up to four days. It's great as a snack—you can dip vegetables in it.

. . . .

PER SERVING: Calories: 262; Total fat: 2g; Saturated fat: <1g; Carbohydrates: 55; Fiber: 8g; Protein: 11g

Crab Salad Sandwiches

QUICK & EASY, MAKE AHEAD **SERVES 2 / PREP TIME: 15 MINUTES**

. . . .

You can make the crab salad up to three days ahead and store it in a tightly sealed container in the refrigerator. You can find canned lump crabmeat in the seafood section of the grocery store. If you are gluten-free, avoid imitation crabmeat (krab) because it contains gluten.

. . . .

½ pound lump crabmeat, drained and picked over

¼ red onion, finely minced

3 tablespoons Greek yogurt

2 tablespoons chopped fresh dill

1 tablespoon Dijon mustard

8 cherry tomatoes, halved

4 slices whole-wheat bread, toasted

1. In a large bowl, mix the crab, onion, yogurt, dill, mustard, and tomatoes.
2. Spread on 2 pieces of toast and cover with the remaining 2.

. . . .

COOKING TIP: Serve this tasty sandwich with one of the salads in this chapter on the side for a delicious meal. Feel free to use gluten-free bread.

. . . .

PER SERVING: Calories: 310; Total fat: 5g; Saturated fat: 1g; Carbohydrates: 39; Fiber: 7g; Protein: 27g

Pesto Chicken Sandwiches

QUICK & EASY SERVES 2 / PREP TIME: 15 MINUTES

. . . .

If you break down a whole rotisserie chicken (removing bones and skin) and store it in zip-top bags in the freezer in 1-cup servings, you save time and have plenty of chicken for weekday meals. You can save even more time by purchasing commercially prepared pesto. However, making your own pesto is quick, easy, and delicious.

. . . .

FOR THE PESTO

2 bunches fresh basil, stems removed

3 tablespoons extra-virgin olive oil

¼ cup grated Parmesan cheese

¼ cup walnuts

FOR THE SANDWICHES

2 cups rotisserie chicken, shredded

3 tablespoons Greek yogurt

¼ cup pesto (above)

4 slices whole-wheat bread, toasted

1 cup baby spinach

TO MAKE THE PESTO

In a food processor, combine all ingredients. Pulse for 20 to 30 one-second pulses, until the nuts are chopped.

TO MAKE THE SANDWICHES

1. In a small bowl, combine the chicken, yogurt, and pesto.
2. Spread on 2 pieces of bread. Top each sandwich with baby spinach and the second slice of bread.

. . . .

COOKING TIP: Leftover pesto stores best in the refrigerator. Put it in an airtight container and store it for up to one week. It will also freeze well in ice cube trays. Freeze and then store the cubes in a zip-top bag.

. . . .

PER SERVING: Calories: 540; Total fat: 21g; Saturated fat: 5g; Carbohydrates: 37; Fiber: 7g; Protein: 50g

Moroccan Veggie and Chickpea
Couscous, page 93

CHAPTER 6

Meatless Mains

Mushroom and Red Wine Ragout with Whole-Wheat Pasta

MAKE AHEAD, LEFTOVERS LUNCH

SERVES 6 / PREP TIME: 15 MINUTES / COOK TIME: 45 MINUTES

Mushrooms are a hearty addition to this flavorful pasta dish. While the recipe calls for whole-wheat pasta, you can also put the ragout on cooked quinoa or steamed brown rice if you would like an equally delicious gluten-free version. Porcini mushrooms add the best flavor here, but you can use any that you'd like.

1 ounce dried mushrooms

2 cups vegetable broth, boiling

3 tablespoons extra-virgin olive oil

1 red onion, finely diced

1 pound cremini mushrooms, sliced

1 pound shiitake mushrooms, sliced

1 teaspoon dried thyme

½ teaspoon sea salt

4 garlic cloves, minced

2 tablespoons flour (substitute gluten-free if needed)

½ cup dry red wine

¼ teaspoon freshly cracked black pepper

3 cups dry whole-wheat rotini pasta, cooked according to package directions and drained

1. In a large heatproof bowl, combine the dried mushrooms and vegetable broth. Cover and allow to sit for 30 minutes.
2. Drain the liquid from the mushrooms, reserving both the mushrooms and the liquid. Finely chop the rehydrated mushrooms.
3. In a large skillet, heat the olive oil on medium-high until it shimmers.
4. Add the red onion and cook, stirring occasionally, until it is transparent, about 4 minutes.
5. Add the fresh and rehydrated mushrooms, thyme, and salt. Cook, stirring occasionally, until the mushrooms are well browned, about 7 minutes.
6. Add the garlic and cook, stirring constantly, for 30 seconds.
7. Add the flour and cook, stirring constantly, for 1 minute.
8. Add the red wine. Use the side of a wooden spoon to scrape any browned bits from the bottom of the pan.
9. Add the reserved liquid from the mushrooms. Bring to a simmer and reduce the heat to medium-low. Add the pepper.

10. Cook, stirring occasionally, until the liquid is thick and gravy-like, 2 to 3 minutes.

11. Serve spooned over the cooked pasta.

....

COOKING TIP: Clean the mushrooms thoroughly before slicing them. To do this, use a dry paper towel or mushroom brush to gently wipe away any loose dirt from the mushrooms. Don't run them under water, which can waterlog them and make the sauce thinner.

....

PER SERVING: Calories: 280; Total fat: 8g; Saturated fat: 1g; Carbohydrates: 45g; Fiber: 6g; Protein: 10g

Pasta Primavera

SERVES 6 / PREP TIME: 15 MINUTES / COOK TIME: 20 MINUTES

. . . .

This light, fresh pasta dish makes a beautiful and colorful meal packed with fresh veggies. The touch of white wine in the sauce adds a luxurious flavor. If you plan to make this ahead, then store the sauce and the pasta separately and reheat just before serving.

. . . .

3 tablespoons extra-virgin olive oil

1 red onion, finely diced

2 carrots, peeled and julienned

2 small zucchini, julienned

1 red bell pepper, seeds and ribs removed, julienned

1 yellow bell pepper, seeds and ribs removed, julienned

1 tablespoon dried Italian herbs

½ teaspoon sea salt

3 garlic cloves, minced

½ cup dry white wine or white wine vinegar

1 pound cherry tomatoes, halved

¼ cup chopped fresh basil

3 cups dry whole-wheat rotini or penne pasta, cooked according to package directions and drained

1. In a large skillet, heat the olive oil on medium-high until it shimmers.
2. Add the red onion, carrots, zucchini, bell peppers, Italian herbs, and salt. Cook, stirring occasionally, until the vegetables are soft, about 7 minutes.
3. Add the garlic and cook, stirring constantly, for 30 seconds.
4. Add the wine and cook, stirring occasionally, until the wine is reduced by half, about 5 minutes.
5. Stir in the tomatoes and cook, stirring for 30 seconds.
6. Remove from the heat and stir in the basil.
7. Serve spooned over the cooked pasta.

. . . .

SUBSTITUTION TIP: If you don't need to cook a vegan meal, you can top this with ½ cup of shredded Parmesan cheese.

. . . .

PER SERVING: Calories: 231; Total fat: 8g; Saturated fat: 1g; Carbohydrates: 33g; Fiber: 6g; Protein: 6g

Rice and Bean Burritos

MAKE AHEAD **SERVES 4 / PREP TIME: 15 MINUTES / COOK TIME: 45 MINUTES**

Using precooked rice and canned black beans makes this recipe quick and easy. You can eat this meal as a lunch, making the burritos ahead of time and reheating in the microwave for 1 to 2 minutes depending on the microwave's power. You can even store the burritos in zip-top bags in the freezer for up to six months.

2 tablespoons extra-virgin olive oil

1 red onion, chopped

1 green bell pepper, seeds and ribs removed, chopped

4 garlic cloves, minced

1 (14-ounce) can low-sodium black beans, drained

1 cup cooked brown rice

1 teaspoon chili powder

½ teaspoon ground cumin

½ teaspoon ground coriander

Juice of 1 lime

½ teaspoon sea salt

4 whole-wheat tortillas

½ cup grated pepper jack cheese (optional)

1. Preheat your oven to 375°F.
2. In a large skillet, heat the olive oil on medium-high until it shimmers.
3. Add the red onion and green pepper and cook, stirring occasionally, until the vegetables are soft, about 5 minutes.
4. Add the garlic and cook, stirring constantly, for 30 seconds.
5. Add the beans, rice, chili powder, cumin, coriander, lime juice, and sea salt. Cook until the rice and beans are heated through, about 4 minutes.
6. Divide the filling evenly among 4 tortillas. Sprinkle with the cheese, if using, and roll into a burrito.
7. Bake on a rimmed baking sheet in the preheated oven for 20 to 30 minutes, until heated through.

COOKING TIP: Serve topped with prepared salsa or prepared guacamole if you wish.

PER SERVING: Calories: 371; Total fat: 11g; Saturated fat: 2g; Carbohydrates: 57g; Fiber: 10g; Protein: 12g

Eggplant, Bell Pepper, and Tomato Bake

LEFTOVERS LUNCH SERVES 8 / PREP TIME: 15 MINUTES / COOK TIME: 45 MINUTES

. . . .

The trick to this eggplant dish is very thin slices of eggplant, which take on a crispier texture. Use a slicer or mandoline and slice them to ¼- to ½-inch thickness. The cheese in this dish is optional; if you don't consume dairy, you can leave it off completely.

. . . .

1½ cups bread crumbs (or gluten-free bread crumbs)

2 large eggs, beaten

1 eggplant, very thinly sliced

2 tablespoons extra-virgin olive oil

½ red onion, finely chopped

1 red bell pepper, seeds and ribs removed, chopped

4 garlic cloves, minced

2 (28-ounce) cans crushed tomatoes, undrained

1 tablespoon dried Italian herbs

½ teaspoon sea salt

Pinch red pepper flakes

4 ounces grated Parmesan cheese

1. Preheat your oven to 400°F.
2. Spread the bread crumbs on a plate.
3. Dip the eggplant slices in the egg and then in the bread crumbs to coat. Place in a single layer on rimmed baking sheets.
4. Bake in the preheated oven for 6 minutes, until the bread crumbs brown. Flip and bake an additional 6 minutes. Remove from the oven and reduce the heat to 375°F.
5. While the eggplant bakes, heat the olive oil in a large skillet on medium-high until it shimmers.
6. Add the onion and red bell pepper and cook, stirring occasionally, until the vegetables are soft, about 5 minutes.
7. Add the garlic and cook, stirring constantly, for 30 seconds.
8. Add the crushed tomatoes, Italian herbs, sea salt, and red pepper flakes. Bring to a simmer. Reduce the heat to medium-low and cook, stirring occasionally, for 10 minutes.
9. In a deep 9-by-13-inch baking pan, spoon a thin layer of sauce over the bottom of the pan.

10. Add a thin layer of eggplant in a single layer. Spoon more sauce on the top and add an additional layer of eggplant. Spoon sauce on the top of that, and add a final layer of eggplant. Spoon the remaining sauce over the top and sprinkle with the cheese.

11. Bake in the preheated oven until bubbly, about 20 minutes.

. . . .

COOKING TIP: You can remove bitter fluids from the eggplant before cooking it by using salt. To do this, place the sliced eggplant in a colander over a bowl and salt it liberally. Let it sit for 30 minutes to allow the fluids to run out of the eggplant. Then, rinse away the salt and use it in the recipe as written.

. . . .

PER SERVING: Calories: 274; Total fat: 9g; Saturated fat: 4g; Carbohydrates: 35g; Fiber: 6g; Protein: 14g

Egg, Veggie, and Parmesan Casserole

MAKE AHEAD, LEFTOVERS LUNCH

SERVES 6 / PREP TIME: 15 MINUTES / COOK TIME: 35 MINUTES

The great thing about this egg casserole is how easy it is to make ahead. You can cut it into single servings and freeze leftovers in zip-top bags for up to six months, then reheat it easily in the microwave. It's versatile enough to be served as breakfast, lunch, or dinner.

Nonstick cooking spray

2 tablespoons extra-virgin olive oil

1 red onion, finely chopped

1 red bell pepper, seeds and ribs removed, chopped

1 cup broccoli florets, cut small

3 garlic cloves, minced

9 large eggs, beaten

½ cup skim milk or nondairy milk

1 tablespoon dried thyme

½ teaspoon sea salt

¼ teaspoon freshly cracked black pepper

1 cup grated Parmesan cheese

1. Preheat your oven to 375°F. Coat a 9-by-13-inch casserole pan with nonstick cooking spray.
2. In a large skillet, heat the olive oil on medium-high until it shimmers.
3. Add the onion, bell pepper, and broccoli and cook, stirring occasionally, until the veggies are soft, 5 to 7 minutes.
4. Add the garlic and cook, stirring constantly, for 30 seconds.
5. Remove from the heat and allow to cool. Spread in an even layer in the bottom of the prepared baking dish.
6. In a large bowl, combine the eggs, milk, thyme, salt, and pepper. Whisk until the eggs are well beaten. Then fold in the cheese.
7. Pour over the vegetables in an even layer.
8. Bake in the preheated oven until the eggs are set, about 25 minutes.

SUBSTITUTION TIP: This is a very adaptable recipe. You can use any veggies you wish here. Try substituting 2 cups of kale, stems removed and chopped, for the broccoli, or try adding a cup of baby spinach.

PER SERVING: Calories: 253; Total fat: 17g; Saturated fat: 6g; Carbohydrates: 7g; Fiber: 1g; Protein: 18g

Three-Bean Chili

ONE POT, MAKE AHEAD, LEFTOVERS LUNCH

SERVES 6 / PREP TIME: 5 MINUTES / COOK TIME: 20 MINUTES

Chili may be the perfect meal. It's delicious at lunch or dinner, it cooks in one pot, and it freezes well for up to six months, so it's easy to make ahead and reheat. If you prefer your chili a little spicier, you can add more cayenne, or omit it altogether for a milder chili.

3 tablespoons extra-virgin olive oil

1 red onion, chopped

1 green bell pepper, seeds and ribs removed, chopped

3 garlic cloves, minced

1 (14-ounce) can low-sodium black beans, drained

1 (14-ounce) can low-sodium kidney beans, drained

1 (14-ounce) can low-sodium pinto beans, drained

1 (28-ounce) can crushed tomatoes, undrained

1 tablespoon chili powder

1 teaspoon ground cumin

½ teaspoon dried oregano

½ cup water or vegetable broth

½ teaspoon sea salt

Dash cayenne pepper

1. In a large pot, heat the olive oil on medium-high until it shimmers.
2. Add the red onion and green pepper and cook, stirring occasionally, until the veggies are soft, about 5 minutes.
3. Add the garlic and cook, stirring constantly, for 30 seconds.
4. Add the beans, tomatoes, chili powder, cumin, oregano, water or broth, salt, and cayenne. Bring to a simmer. Reduce the heat to medium-low. Cook, stirring occasionally, for 10 minutes more.

SUBSTITUTION TIP: While three different kinds of beans add different flavors and textures to this chili, you can also use just a single type of any of the beans listed here.

PER SERVING: Calories: 302; Total fat: 7g; Saturated fat: 1g; Carbohydrates: 44g; Fiber: 12g; Protein: 14g

Quick Tofu and Veggie Stir-Fry

QUICK & EASY, ONE POT, LEFTOVERS LUNCH

SERVES 6 / PREP TIME: 15 MINUTES / COOK TIME: 15 MINUTES

. . . .

This recipe calls for extra-firm tofu, which works best for cooking in stir-fries. Tofu is a great source of protein that turns this vegetarian dish into a hearty meal. If you want it to hold sauce better, try tearing the tofu into bite-size pieces rather than chopping.

. . . .

3 tablespoons extra-virgin olive oil, divided

1 (14-ounce) block extra-firm tofu, cut into ¾-inch pieces

2 tablespoons low-sodium soy sauce (or tamari soy sauce for gluten-free), divided

1 bunch green onions, sliced

1 cup broccoli florets, chopped

1 red bell pepper, seeds and ribs removed, chopped

1 cup sliced shiitake mushrooms

2 garlic cloves, minced

1 tablespoon freshly grated ginger

1 tablespoon apple cider vinegar

Juice of 1 lime

½ teaspoon sriracha

¼ teaspoon sesame oil

1 teaspoon cornstarch

¼ cup fresh chopped cilantro

1½ cups cooked brown rice

1. In a large skillet or wok, heat 1 tablespoon of olive oil on medium-high until it shimmers.
2. Add the tofu and drizzle with 1 tablespoon of soy sauce. Cook, stirring occasionally, until the tofu is browned, about 5 minutes. Remove from the pan and set aside.
3. Add the remaining 2 tablespoons of olive oil to the pan and heat until it shimmers.
4. Add the green onions, broccoli, bell pepper, and mushrooms. Cook, stirring occasionally, until the veggies soften and begin to brown, 5 to 7 minutes.
5. Add the garlic and cook, stirring constantly, for 30 seconds.
6. In a small bowl, whisk together the remaining 1 tablespoon of soy sauce and the ginger, vinegar, lime juice, sriracha, sesame oil, and cornstarch.
7. Return the tofu to the pan and add the sauce. Cook, stirring, until the sauce thickens, about 3 minutes more.
8. Remove from heat and stir in the cilantro. Serve over the cooked rice.

. . . .

COOKING TIP: To get the tofu crispy, press out some of the water. To do this, wrap the whole block of tofu in paper towels, place it on a plate, and cover it with another plate. Weight the top plate with a can or two and allow it to sit while you prep your other veggies, or for about 15 minutes.

. . . .

PER SERVING: Calories: 217; Total fat: 11g; Saturated fat: 2g; Carbohydrates: 22g; Fiber: 4g; Protein: 9g

Moroccan Veggie and Chickpea Couscous

QUICK & EASY **SERVES 4 / PREP TIME: 15 MINUTES / COOK TIME: 15 MINUTES**

Couscous is a North African staple food. It's so easy to make, and it's a delicious grain base for this veggie and chickpea dish. Using whole-wheat couscous increases fiber but doesn't take any longer to cook or prepare than a traditional white couscous.

¾ cup whole-wheat couscous

3 tablespoons extra-virgin olive oil, divided

3 cups low-sodium vegetable broth, boiling, divided

1 red onion, thinly sliced

1 small eggplant, chopped into ½-inch pieces

1 red bell pepper, seeds and ribs removed, chopped

4 garlic cloves, minced

1 (14-ounce) can low-sodium chickpeas, drained

1 teaspoon freshly grated ginger

1 teaspoon ground cumin

¼ teaspoon ground allspice

¼ teaspoon ground coriander

½ teaspoon sea salt

¼ teaspoon freshly cracked black pepper

1. Put the couscous in a large, heatproof bowl. Add 1 tablespoon of olive oil and toss to coat.
2. Pour 1½ cups of boiling vegetable broth over the top of the couscous. Cover and allow it to sit while you prepare the other ingredients.
3. In a large skillet, heat the remaining 2 tablespoons of olive oil on medium-high until it shimmers.
4. Add the onion, eggplant, and bell pepper. Cook, stirring occasionally, until the vegetables soften, about 5 minutes.
5. Add the garlic and cook, stirring constantly, for 30 seconds.
6. Add the remaining 1½ cups of broth and the chickpeas, ginger, cumin, allspice, coriander, salt, and pepper. Bring to a simmer and reduce the heat to medium-low.
7. Cook, stirring, for 5 minutes.
8. Fluff the couscous with a fork, then add to the skillet. Cook, stirring, for 2 minutes more.

COOKING TIP: To reduce the bitterness of the eggplant, put the cut pieces in a colander over the sink or a bowl, salt them, and allow them to sit for 20 minutes before using. Then, rinse the salt away from the eggplant and pat it dry before adding it to the dish.

PER SERVING: Calories: 397; Total fat: 13g; Saturated fat: 2g; Carbohydrates: 63g; Fiber: 14g; Protein: 13g

Broccoli, Kale, and Quinoa Bowl

LEFTOVERS LUNCH **SERVES 6 / PREP TIME: 10 MINUTES / COOK TIME: 30 MINUTES**

If you plan ahead, you can cook larger quantities of quinoa ahead of time following steps 1 and 2 and freeze it in one-cup servings. Thaw in the microwave, and you'll be ready to make this quick and easy one-pot dish that's packed with cruciferous goodness. You can also use cooked brown rice if you wish.

2 tablespoons plus 1 teaspoon extra-virgin olive oil, divided

1 cup quinoa, rinsed

1¾ cups low-sodium vegetable broth

1 red onion, chopped

2 cups broccoli florets, chopped

2 cups kale, stems removed, chopped

1 red bell pepper, seeds and ribs removed, chopped

1 tablespoon freshly grated ginger

3 garlic cloves, minced

1 tablespoon low-sodium soy sauce (or tamari for gluten-free)

½ teaspoon sriracha

½ cup chopped peanuts or almonds

1. In a small saucepan over medium heat, heat 1 teaspoon of olive oil on medium-high until it shimmers. Add the quinoa and toast, stirring, for 2 minutes.
2. Add the vegetable broth. Bring to a boil. Reduce heat to medium-low. Cover and cook for 20 minutes. Remove from the heat and allow it to stand, covered, for 5 minutes more. Fluff with a fork.
3. While the quinoa cooks, heat the remaining 2 tablespoons of olive oil in a large skillet on medium-high until it shimmers.
4. Add the onion, broccoli, kale, bell pepper, and ginger. Cook, stirring occasionally, until the vegetables soften, about 7 minutes.
5. Add the garlic and cook, stirring constantly, for 30 seconds.
6. Add the soy sauce, sriracha, and cooked quinoa. Cook to heat through, stirring, about 4 minutes more.
7. Remove from heat and top with the chopped nuts.

COOKING TIP: Don't skip the step of rinsing the quinoa. It removes bitter flavors and results in a much tastier dish. To rinse, put the quinoa in a fine-mesh sieve and run it under cold water, rubbing the grains of quinoa with your fingers as you do. Rinse until the water runs clear.

PER SERVING: Calories: 260; Total fat: 12g; Saturated fat: 2g; Carbohydrates: 31g; Fiber: 5g; Protein: 8g

Quick Sweet Potato and Vegetable Curry

ONE POT, MAKE AHEAD, LEFTOVERS LUNCH

SERVES 6 / PREP TIME: 10 MINUTES / COOK TIME: 20 MINUTES

Curry makes a hearty and warming meal by itself or served over rice or quinoa. As it rests in the refrigerator over a day or two, the flavors blend together even better. That makes this curry the perfect make-ahead meal, leaving you with leftovers that will travel well for tomorrow's lunch.

2 tablespoons extra-virgin olive oil

1 tablespoon freshly grated ginger

2 garlic cloves, minced

2 tablespoons curry powder

2 sweet potatoes, peeled and cut into ¾-inch cubes

1 (14-ounce) can low-sodium chickpeas, drained

4 cups baby spinach

½ cup low-sodium vegetable broth

1 (14-ounce) can light coconut milk

½ teaspoon sea salt

Juice of 1 lime

1. In a large pot, heat the olive oil on medium-high until it shimmers. Add the ginger, garlic, and curry powder and cook, stirring, for 1 minute.
2. Add the sweet potatoes, chickpeas, spinach, vegetable broth, coconut milk, and salt. Bring to a simmer. Reduce the heat to medium-low.
3. Cook, stirring occasionally, until the sweet potatoes soften, 10 to 15 minutes.
4. Remove from heat and stir in the lime juice.

SUBSTITUTION TIP: This curry lends itself well to the addition of more veggies if you like. Add up to 1 cup each of chopped broccoli florets and chopped kale with the stems removed to bring in more cruciferous vegetables.

PER SERVING: Calories: 216; Total fat: 10g; Saturated fat: 4g; Carbohydrates: 27g; Fiber: 6g; Protein: 6g

Oven-Baked Chicken and Veggie Kebabs, page 110

CHAPTER 7

Poultry, Fish & Seafood

Cod and Veggies in Parchment

QUICK & EASY SERVES 4 / PREP TIME: 10 MINUTES / COOK TIME: 15 MINUTES

Cooking fish in parchment paper helps it stay moist, resulting in fish with a delicate texture. If you don't have parchment paper, you can also create sealed foil packets, which will have the same effect on the fish and veggies. Feel free to substitute any white fish or even trout or salmon for the cod.

4 squares of parchment paper or foil large enough to wrap fish and veggies

4 (4-ounce) cod fillets

½ teaspoon sea salt

¼ teaspoon freshly cracked black pepper

1 teaspoon dried dill

4 lemon slices

1 red bell pepper, seeds and ribs removed, thinly sliced

½ red onion, thinly sliced

1 small zucchini, cut into thin strips using a vegetable peeler

4 tablespoons extra-virgin olive oil

1 cup dry white wine or white wine vinegar

1. Preheat your oven to 400°F.
2. Place a piece of cod in the center of each piece of parchment paper.
3. Season each piece of cod with the salt, pepper, and dill and top each with a lemon slice.
4. Evenly distribute the bell pepper, onion, and zucchini on top of each piece of cod.
5. Drizzle 1 tablespoon of olive oil over each.
6. Fold the parchment paper around the fish and vegetables, leaving the top unsealed.
7. Carefully pour ¼ cup of dry white wine into each packet and then fold the packet to seal it.
8. Place the packets on a rimmed baking sheet and put it in the preheated oven.
9. Bake until the fish is flaky and the vegetables soft, about 15 minutes.

SUBSTITUTION TIP: If you're not a fan of fish, or if you're allergic to fish (but not shellfish), you can replace the cod with 4 ounces of prawns.

PER SERVING: Calories: 303; Total fat: 15g; Saturated fat: 2g; Carbohydrates: 8g; Fiber: 2g; Protein: 27g

Scallops with Citrus Spinach

QUICK & EASY SERVES 4 / PREP TIME: 10 MINUTES / COOK TIME: 10 MINUTES

Use large sea scallops for this recipe, not small bay scallops. If you're purchasing frozen scallops rather than fresh, place the bag of frozen scallops in a bowl of cold water to thaw, changing the water every 15 minutes. The scallops will take about an hour to thaw completely.

4 tablespoons extra-virgin olive oil, divided

1 pound sea scallops

½ teaspoon sea salt, divided

¼ teaspoon freshly cracked black pepper, divided

5 cups baby spinach

Juice of 1 lemon

Juice of 1 lime

1. In a large skillet, heat 2 tablespoons of olive oil on medium-high until it shimmers.
2. Season the scallops with ¼ teaspoon of salt and ⅛ teaspoon of pepper.
3. Place the scallops in the hot oil and cook without moving them until they are seared on one side, about 2 minutes.
4. Use tongs to flip the scallops. Cook without moving until they are seared on the other side, about 2 minutes more.
5. Set the scallops aside on a plate and add the remaining 2 tablespoons of olive oil to the pan. Heat until it shimmers.
6. Add the spinach. Cook, stirring, for 1 minute.
7. Add the lemon and lime juices and the remaining ¼ teaspoon of salt and ⅛ teaspoon of pepper.
8. Cook for 2 minutes more. Place scallops atop the spinach to serve.

COOKING TIP: To prepare the scallops, use a sharp knife to cut away the tendon along the side of the scallop. Then, pat the scallops dry with a paper towel to ensure a nice crust when you sear the scallops.

PER SERVING: Calories: 238; Total fat: 15g; Saturated fat: 2g; Carbohydrates: 5g; Fiber: 1g; Protein: 20g

Shrimp Fried Rice

ONE POT, MAKE AHEAD, LEFTOVERS LUNCH

SERVES 6 / PREP TIME: 10 MINUTES / COOK TIME: 15 MINUTES

This recipe is especially quick and easy because it uses precooked brown rice, either homemade by you in a large batch and frozen in zip-top bags or prepared at the grocery store. The texture of the dish is best if the rice has been allowed to cool before it's added to the skillet. Aside from being easy, the dish features antioxidant-rich carrot and anti-inflammatory ginger.

4 tablespoons extra-virgin olive oil, divided

1 pound shrimp, peeled, deveined, and tails off

1 bunch green onions, sliced

1 carrot, peeled and cut into ¼-inch cubes

1 cup fresh or frozen peas (thawed)

1 tablespoon freshly grated ginger

4 garlic cloves, minced

2 large eggs, beaten

1 tablespoon low-sodium soy sauce (or tamari)

3 cups cooked brown rice

1. In a large skillet, heat 2 tablespoons of olive oil on medium-high until it shimmers.
2. Add the shrimp and cook, stirring, until it is pink, about 4 minutes.
3. Remove the shrimp from the pan and set it aside on a platter.
4. Add the remaining 2 tablespoons of oil to the pan. Heat until it shimmers.
5. Add the green onions, carrots, peas, and ginger. Cook, stirring, until the vegetables soften, about 4 minutes.
6. Add the garlic and cook, stirring constantly, for 30 seconds.
7. Add the eggs and cook, scrambling the eggs until they cook through, about 2 minutes more.
8. Add the soy sauce, rice, and reserved shrimp. Cook, stirring, until the rice heats through, about 3 minutes more.

SUBSTITUTION TIP: You can add other veggies to this rice. For example, add 1 cup of chopped broccoli florets or chopped kale to bring some cruciferous veggies into the mix.

PER SERVING: Calories: 324; Total fat: 13g; Saturated fat: 2g; Carbohydrates: 30g; Fiber: 4g; Protein: 21g

Farfalle with Anchovy Puttanesca

LEFTOVERS LUNCH **SERVES 6 / PREP TIME: 10 MINUTES / COOK TIME: 30 MINUTES**

Puttanesca is a deeply flavorful sauce that's delicious on pasta. You could also use it to top fish or even poultry. If you use this for leftovers at lunch, store the sauce and the pasta separately, and add the sauce to the pasta just before serving.

3 tablespoons extra-virgin olive oil

6 anchovy fillets, chopped

4 garlic cloves, sliced

¼ teaspoon red pepper flakes

2 tablespoons tomato paste

1 (35-ounce) can crushed tomatoes, undrained

1 tablespoon dried Italian herbs

¼ cup chopped black olives

1 tablespoon capers, drained

12 ounces whole-wheat farfalle pasta, cooked according to package directions and drained

1. In a large skillet, heat the olive oil on medium until it shimmers.
2. Add the anchovies, garlic, and red pepper flakes. Cook, stirring, until the anchovies are golden, about 5 minutes.
3. Add the tomato paste. Cook, stirring, for 1 minute.
4. Add the crushed tomatoes, Italian herbs, olives, and capers. Bring to a boil. Reduce the heat to medium-low and simmer, stirring, until the sauce thickens, about 20 minutes.
5. Serve spooned over the hot pasta.

SUBSTITUTION TIP: For more Italian flavor, use an equal amount of canned Italian tomatoes with basil in place of the crushed tomatoes. If the tomatoes are whole, crush them with your hands before adding them. You can also add fresh flavors by stirring in ¼ cup chopped fresh basil or chopped fresh Italian parsley after you've removed the sauce from the heat.

PER SERVING: Calories: 340; Total fat: 9g; Saturated fat: 1g; Carbohydrates: 48g; Fiber: 10g; Protein: 13g

Salmon with Blackberry Glaze

QUICK & EASY SERVES 4 / PREP TIME: 10 MINUTES / COOK TIME: 20 MINUTES

Salmon has rich red flesh that holds up well to the sweet flavors of blackberry. This delicious salmon is tasty with a simple side salad, some steamed veggies, or a side of brown rice or quinoa. You can also grill the salmon outdoors on your barbecue for a lovely summer meal.

4 tablespoons extra-virgin olive oil, divided

4 (4-ounce) salmon fillets

½ teaspoon sea salt

¼ teaspoon freshly cracked black pepper

2 tablespoons minced shallots

Juice of 1 orange

2 cups blackberries

1 teaspoon dried thyme

Pinch red pepper flakes

1. In a large skillet, heat 2 tablespoons of olive oil on medium-high until it shimmers.
2. Season the salmon with salt and pepper.
3. Place the salmon, skin-side up, in the hot oil and cook without moving for 4 minutes.
4. Flip the salmon and cook until the skin is crisp, about 3 minutes.
5. Remove the salmon from the pan and set it aside on a plate tented with foil. Return the pan to the heat.
6. Add the remaining 2 tablespoons of olive oil. Add the shallots and cook, stirring occasionally, until soft, about 3 minutes.
7. Add the orange juice, blackberries, thyme, and red pepper flakes. Cook, stirring occasionally and crushing the berries, until the mixture thickens slightly, about 4 minutes.
8. Serve with the sauce spooned over the top of the salmon.

COOKING TIP: Prepare the salmon by removing the pin bones. Use small needle-nose pliers or tweezers to remove the bones.

PER SERVING: Calories: 305; Total fat: 19g; Saturated fat: 3g; Carbohydrates: 11g; Fiber: 4g; Protein: 24g

Maple and Citrus–Glazed Salmon

QUICK & EASY **SERVES 4 / PREP TIME: 15 MINUTES / COOK TIME: 10 MINUTES**

Maple and orange beautifully complement the slightly sweet flavor of salmon. This is a very fast and easy recipe, so it's perfect for a busy weeknight when you only have a few minutes to cook. Add a side salad, and you've got a well-balanced, flavorful meal.

2 tablespoons low-sodium soy sauce (or tamari for gluten-free)

¼ cup pure maple syrup

Juice of 2 oranges

4 (4-ounce) salmon fillets

2 tablespoons extra-virgin olive oil

¼ teaspoon freshly cracked black pepper

1. In a shallow dish, whisk together the soy sauce, syrup, and orange juice.
2. Place the salmon fillets flesh-side down in the marinade and allow to sit for 10 minutes.
3. In a large skillet, heat the olive oil on medium-high until it shimmers.
4. Remove the salmon from the marinade and pat it dry with a paper towel. Season with the pepper.
5. Place the salmon skin-side up in the hot oil and cook without moving for 4 minutes.
6. Flip the salmon and cook until the skin is crisp, about 3 minutes.

ON THE MENU: Serve this with the Spinach and Strawberry Salad found on page 72, or the Red Cabbage, Ginger, and Apple Asian Slaw on page 73.

PER SERVING: Calories: 270; Total fat: 12g; Saturated fat: 2g; Carbohydrates: 17g; Fiber: <1g; Protein: 24g

Mediterranean Salmon Burgers with Tzatziki

SERVES 4 / PREP TIME: 15 MINUTES, PLUS 30 MINUTES TO REST / COOK TIME: 15 MINUTES

Make burger night more interesting with these Mediterranean-spiced salmon burgers with fresh veggies and homemade tzatziki sauce. It's a delicious take on a salmon burger with lots of flavor. Use leftover sauce for dipping vegetables, or spread it on bread.

1 (15-ounce) can wild caught salmon, drained

¼ cup crumbled feta cheese

¼ cup whole-wheat bread crumbs

1 large egg, beaten

2 tablespoons finely minced shallot

2 cloves garlic, minced, divided

1 teaspoon dried dill

1 teaspoon ground coriander

½ teaspoon cumin

½ teaspoon sea salt, plus more for seasoning

½ cup plain Greek yogurt

½ cup grated cucumber

¼ cup grated red onion, plus 4 red onion slices, divided

1 teaspoon freshly squeezed lemon juice

2 tablespoons extra-virgin olive oil

4 whole-wheat hamburger buns, toasted

4 tomato slices

1. In a medium bowl, combine the salmon, feta, bread crumbs, egg, shallot, 1 clove of minced garlic, dill, coriander, cumin, and ½ teaspoon salt. Mix well. Form into 4 patties and refrigerate for at least 30 minutes.

2. Make the tzatziki by mixing together the Greek yogurt, cucumber, grated red onion, remaining 1 clove of minced garlic, lemon juice, and a pinch salt in a small bowl. Set aside.

3. In a large, nonstick skillet, heat the olive oil on medium-high until it shimmers.

4. Add the salmon patties and cook until browned on both sides, about 5 minutes per side.

5. Place the patties on the buns. Top with the tzatziki sauce, tomato slices, and red onion slices.

SUBSTITUTION TIP: To make this gluten-free, replace the bread crumbs with ¼ cup of almond meal and replace the hamburger buns with gluten-free buns, gluten-free bread, or lettuce wraps.

PER SERVING: Calories: 453; Total fat: 22g; Saturated fat: 6g; Carbohydrates: 35g; Fiber: 5g; Protein: 33g

Quick Turkey Piccata

QUICK & EASY SERVES 4 / PREP TIME: 10 MINUTES / COOK TIME: 15 MINUTES

This lemony, briny Italian dish cooks quickly because you'll be pounding the turkey breasts very thin. You could serve this with steamed asparagus and cooked quinoa to make a delicious dinner. The piccata also works alongside a side salad for a lighter lunch.

½ cup flour

½ teaspoon sea salt

¼ teaspoon freshly cracked black pepper

1 pound turkey tenders, pounded to ⅛-inch thickness (see Cooking Tip)

4 tablespoons extra-virgin olive oil, divided

2 tablespoons minced shallot

2 garlic cloves, minced

½ cup dry white wine

Juice of 1 lemon

1 tablespoon capers, drained and rinsed

2 tablespoons very cold unsalted butter, cut into pieces

¼ cup chopped fresh Italian parsley

1. In a shallow dish, whisk together the flour, salt, and pepper.
2. Dip the turkey pieces in the flour mixture and tap off any excess.
3. In a large skillet, heat 2 tablespoons of olive oil on medium-high until it shimmers.
4. Add the turkey and cook without moving before flipping until golden brown on both sides, about 2 minutes per side. Remove from the pan and set aside on a plate tented with foil to keep warm.
5. In the same pan, add the remaining 2 tablespoons of olive oil. Heat until it shimmers.
6. Add the shallot and cook until soft, about 3 minutes.
7. Add the garlic and cook, stirring, for 30 seconds.
8. Add the white wine, lemon juice, and capers, using the side of the spoon to scrape any browned bits from the bottom of the pan. Bring to a simmer.
9. Reduce the heat to low. Simmer until the liquid is reduced by half, about 3 minutes.
10. Whisk in the butter 1 piece at a time until melted.
11. Return the turkey to the pan, turning it in the sauce to coat. Serve and garnish with the parsley.

COOKING TIP: To pound the turkey, place turkey tenders between two pieces of plastic wrap and pound with a mallet into ⅛-inch thickness.

PER SERVING: Calories: 372; Total fat: 20g; Saturated fat: 6g; Carbohydrates: 14g; Fiber: 1g; Protein: 30g

Pasta Carbonara with Peas

QUICK & EASY **SERVES 4 / PREP TIME: 10 MINUTES / COOK TIME: 20 MINUTES**

Carbonara is essentially a rich, cheesy bacon-and-egg pasta, usually made with spaghetti. This recipe uses turkey bacon to cut down on saturated fat without sacrificing flavor. You can use fresh or frozen peas in the recipe, although fresh have a slightly better texture.

2 tablespoons extra-virgin olive oil

6 slices turkey bacon, cut into bite-size pieces

2 tablespoons minced shallot

2 cups fresh or frozen (thawed) peas

3 garlic cloves, minced

8 ounces whole-wheat spaghetti, cooked according to package instructions and drained

6 large eggs, beaten

2 tablespoons skim milk

½ cup grated Parmesan cheese

½ teaspoon sea salt

¼ teaspoon freshly cracked black pepper

Pinch red pepper flakes

1. In a large skillet, heat the olive oil on medium-high until it shimmers.
2. Add the bacon and cook, stirring occasionally, until browned, about 5 minutes.
3. Add the shallot and peas and cook until soft, about 3 minutes.
4. Add the garlic and cook, stirring, for 30 seconds.
5. Add the hot pasta and stir to mix. Remove from the heat.
6. In a small bowl, beat together the eggs, milk, cheese, salt, black pepper, and red pepper flakes.
7. Pour the egg mixture in a thin stream into the pan (off-heat) with the pasta-and-bacon mixture. Stir until the eggs thicken slightly.

COOKING TIP: If you prefer a spicier carbonara, you can add up to ½ teaspoon of red pepper flakes, depending on how much heat you want.

PER SERVING: Calories: 556; Total fat: 22g; Saturated fat: 6g; Carbohydrates: 55g; Fiber: 9g; Protein: 35g

Spaghetti with Turkey Meatballs

MAKE AHEAD, LEFTOVERS LUNCH

SERVES 6 / PREP TIME: 20 MINUTES / COOK TIME: 30 MINUTES

. . . .

This is a great make-ahead recipe. Whenever you have time, you can make a batch of meatballs and sauce and freeze them separately in single-serving containers. Once you have these ready to go in your freezer, you can thaw them and add them to cooked pasta anytime you need a quick meal.

. . . .

FOR THE MEATBALLS

1 pound ground turkey breast

½ cup bread crumbs

½ red onion, minced

4 garlic cloves, minced

1 large egg, beaten

1 tablespoon dried Italian herbs

Pinch red pepper flakes

½ teaspoon sea salt

⅛ teaspoon freshly cracked black pepper

2 tablespoons extra-virgin olive oil

TO MAKE THE MEATBALLS

1. In a large bowl, combine the turkey breast, bread crumbs, onion, garlic, egg, Italian herbs, red pepper flakes, salt, and black pepper.
2. Roll into ½-inch meatballs.
3. In a large pot, heat the olive oil on medium-high until it shimmers. Working in batches, cook the meatballs in the hot oil until cooked through, about 7 minutes.
4. Set aside on a plate.

CONTINUED ▶

FOR THE PASTA AND SAUCE

2 tablespoons extra-virgin olive oil

½ red onion, minced

6 garlic cloves, minced

3 (14-ounce) cans crushed tomatoes, undrained

2 tablespoons dried Italian herbs

½ teaspoon sea salt

¼ teaspoon red pepper flakes

¼ cup chopped fresh basil

12 ounces spaghetti, cooked according to package instructions and drained

TO MAKE THE PASTA AND SAUCE

1. Return the pot you used to cook the meatballs to the stove. Add the olive oil and heat on medium-high until it shimmers.
2. Add the red onion and cook, stirring occasionally, until soft, about 3 minutes.
3. Add the garlic and cook, stirring constantly, for 30 seconds.
4. Add the crushed tomatoes, Italian herbs, salt, and red pepper flakes. Bring to a simmer. Reduce the heat to medium-low and simmer, stirring occasionally, for 10 minutes.
5. Add the meatballs to the sauce and bring to a simmer. Cook for 5 minutes more.
6. Remove from heat and stir in the basil.
7. Serve spooned over the cooked spaghetti.

SUBSTITUTION TIP: Make this gluten-free by replacing the bread crumbs with an equal amount of almond meal and replacing the spaghetti with a gluten-free pasta or zucchini noodles.

PER SERVING: Calories: 493; Total fat: 17g; Saturated fat: 3g; Carbohydrates: 59g; Fiber: 9g; Protein: 26g

Orange Chicken and Quinoa Bowl

LEFTOVERS LUNCH SERVES 6 / PREP TIME: 10 MINUTES / COOK TIME: 30 MINUTES

This zesty chicken dish has a thick, flavorful sauce that comes together in just a few minutes. You can save time by cooking a large batch of quinoa in advance and storing it in zip-top bags in the freezer. Replace 1 cup of dry quinoa with 3 cups of cooked quinoa.

2 tablespoons plus 1 teaspoon extra-virgin olive oil, divided

1 cup quinoa, rinsed

2 cups low-sodium chicken broth, boiling

½ teaspoon sea salt

1 pound boneless, skinless chicken breast, cut into ½-inch pieces

1 red onion, chopped

1 cup broccoli florets

2 cups kale, stems removed and chopped

Juice of 2 oranges and zest of 1 orange

1 tablespoon low-sodium soy sauce

½ teaspoon sriracha

1 teaspoon freshly grated ginger

2 garlic cloves, minced

2 teaspoons cornstarch

1. In a medium pot, heat 1 teaspoon of olive oil on medium-high until it shimmers. Add the quinoa and cook, stirring, for 1 minute. Add the chicken broth and salt and bring to a simmer. Reduce the heat to low, cover, and cook for 15 minutes.

2. Remove from the heat and allow to sit, covered, for 5 minutes more. Fluff with a fork.

3. In a large, nonstick skillet, heat the remaining 2 tablespoons of olive oil on medium-high until it shimmers.

4. Add the chicken and cook, stirring occasionally, until browned, about 5 minutes. Remove the chicken from the pan and set it aside.

5. To the same pan, add the onion, broccoli, and kale. Cook, stirring occasionally, until the vegetables soften and begin to brown, about 5 minutes more.

6. Return the chicken to the pan.

7. In a small bowl, whisk together the orange juice and zest, soy sauce, sriracha, ginger, garlic, and cornstarch.

8. Add to the pan. Cook, stirring, until the sauce thickens, about 4 minutes more.

9. Serve in a bowl spooned over the quinoa.

THE GOOD STUFF: This is an OA powerhouse meal with diallyl disulfide from the garlic and onions plus quercetin and sulforaphane from the cruciferous veggies and red onions.

PER SERVING: Calories: 274; Total fat: 9g; Saturated fat: 1g; Carbohydrates: 28g; Fiber: 4g; Protein: 21g

Oven-Baked Chicken and Veggie Kebabs

SERVES 6 / PREP TIME: 10 MINUTES, PLUS 6 TO 8 HOURS TO MARINATE / COOK TIME: 30 MINUTES

While this recipe calls for baking in the oven, you can also make these chicken and veggie skewers on the grill on sunny summer days. Feel free to use different veggies to create your own twist on a delicious classic. Marinate the chicken in the morning so it's ready to go for dinner in the evening.

1 tablespoon low-sodium soy sauce (or tamari for gluten-free)

Juice of 1 orange

1 teaspoon garlic powder

1 teaspoon onion powder

1 teaspoon Dijon mustard

2 tablespoons extra-virgin olive oil

1½ pounds boneless, skinless chicken breast, cut into 1-inch pieces

12 wooden skewers, soaked in water for 30 minutes

1 pint cherry tomatoes

1 red onion, cut into ½-inch pieces

2 red bell peppers, seeds and ribs removed, cut into ½-inch pieces

2 small zucchini, cut into ½-inch pieces

1. In a medium bowl, combine the soy sauce, orange juice, garlic powder, onion powder, Dijon mustard, and olive oil.
2. Add the chicken pieces and stir to coat. Marinate in the refrigerator for 6 to 8 hours.
3. Preheat your oven to 450°F.
4. Thread the skewers with the chicken, tomatoes, onion, bell peppers, and zucchini. Place on a rimmed baking sheet.
5. Bake for 15 minutes. Turn the skewers and bake another 15 minutes.

COOKING TIP: If grilling, brush the grill with olive oil. Cook about 7 to 10 minutes per side.

PER SERVING: Calories: 194; Total fat: 8g; Saturated fat: 1g; Carbohydrates: 10g; Fiber: 2g; Protein: 25g

Caprese Chicken

QUICK & EASY **SERVES 6 / PREP TIME: 10 MINUTES / COOK TIME: 15 MINUTES**

This simple dinner is delicious with a salad, in a sandwich, or by itself as a delicious main course. Grilling the chicken doesn't take long, and there's no extra time required to marinate. It's especially delicious in the late summer when tomatoes and fresh basil are in season.

4 boneless, skinless chicken breast halves

2 tablespoons extra-virgin olive oil

½ teaspoon sea salt

¼ teaspoon freshly cracked black pepper

1 tablespoon dried Italian herbs

4 (1-ounce) slices mozzarella cheese

4 tomato slices

¼ cup chopped fresh basil

¼ cup balsamic vinegar

1. Preheat a grill or grill pan on high heat.
2. Brush the chicken breasts with the olive oil and season them with the salt, pepper, and Italian herbs.
3. Grill on the preheated grill until cooked through, about 5 minutes per side.
4. With the chicken still on the heat, place 1 slice of mozzarella on each piece of chicken. Cover and cook for 1 minute to slightly melt the cheese.
5. Remove from the heat. Top with the tomato and chopped basil. Drizzle with the balsamic vinegar.

COOKING TIP: To encourage the chicken to cook evenly, place breasts between two pieces of plastic wrap and pound lightly until they are an even thickness.

PER SERVING: Calories: 159; Total fat: 9g; Saturated fat: 3g; Carbohydrates: 3g; Fiber: 1g; Protein: 18g

Baked Chicken Fingers with Honey-and-Garlic Dipping Sauce

QUICK & EASY **SERVES 4 / PREP TIME: 10 MINUTES / COOK TIME: 20 MINUTES**

Baked chicken fingers are a good stand-in for fried chicken. The dish has the crunch and the taste of fried chicken without all the fat, and a garlic dipping sauce adds plenty of flavor. Serve this with a baked sweet potato and steamed veggies for a simple, balanced meal.

FOR THE CHICKEN FINGERS

Nonstick cooking spray

1½ cups bread crumbs

½ teaspoon sea salt

¼ teaspoon freshly cracked black pepper

¼ cup grated Parmesan cheese

2 teaspoons dried thyme

2 large eggs, beaten

1 teaspoon Dijon mustard

1 pound chicken breast tenders

FOR THE DIPPING SAUCE

2 tablespoons olive oil mayonnaise

¼ cup nonfat Greek yogurt

3 garlic cloves, minced

1 tablespoon honey

Pinch sea salt

TO MAKE THE CHICKEN FINGERS

1. Preheat your oven to 400°F. Spray a rimmed baking sheet with nonstick cooking spray.
2. In a medium dish, toss together the bread crumbs, sea salt, pepper, cheese, and thyme.
3. In another bowl, whisk together the eggs and mustard.
4. Dip the chicken in the egg mixture and then into the bread crumb mixture and place on the prepared baking sheet.
5. Bake in the preheated oven until golden, about 20 minutes.

TO MAKE THE DIPPING SAUCE

Whisk together the mayonnaise, yogurt, garlic, and honey in a small bowl. Season with a pinch of salt. Serve as a dipping sauce.

COOKING TIP: If you want your bread crumbs to be even crispier, spritz the coated chicken with a bit of olive oil or cooking spray before you put it in the oven.

PER SERVING: Calories: 375; Total fat: 10g; Saturated fat: 3g; Carbohydrates: 34g; Fiber: 2g; Protein: 36g

Roasted Chicken Thighs with Tomatoes and Olives

ONE POT, LEFTOVERS LUNCH **SERVES 6 / PREP TIME: 10 MINUTES / COOK TIME: 50 MINUTES**

This chicken has complex flavor without requiring much cleanup or active cooking time at all. The chicken thighs and vegetables roast together in one baking pan. You can find the Spanish olives of your choice in the deli section at most grocery stores.

6 chicken thighs

1 red onion, roughly chopped

1 pint cherry tomatoes

½ cup pitted Spanish olives

2 tablespoons extra-virgin olive oil

½ teaspoon sea salt

¼ teaspoon freshly cracked black pepper

1 teaspoon dried thyme

1 teaspoon dried rosemary

¼ cup crumbled feta cheese

1. Preheat your oven to 375°F.
2. In a 9-by-13-inch baking pan, arrange the chicken thighs, onion, tomatoes, and olives.
3. Drizzle with the olive oil and sprinkle with the salt, pepper, thyme, and rosemary.
4. Bake in the preheated oven until the chicken thighs reach a temperature of 165°F, 45 to 50 minutes.
5. Serve topped with feta.

THE GOOD STUFF: Both olives and olive oil are a rich source of oleocanthal, which can help alleviate osteoarthritis symptoms.

PER SERVING: Calories: 332; Total fat: 27g; Saturated fat: 7g; Carbohydrates: 3g; Fiber: 1g; Protein: 20g

Balsamic-Glazed Pork Tenderloin, page 120

CHAPTER 8

Beef, Pork & Lamb

Italian Burgers with Garlic Mayo and Red Onion Quick Pickle

LEFTOVERS LUNCH SERVES 6 / PREP TIME: 15 MINUTES, PLUS 30 MINUTES RESTING TIME / COOK TIME: 20 MINUTES

The trick to pickling red onion is to create very thin slices. The red onion quick pickle adds bright acidity to these rich and flavorful burgers. Store all leftover components separately in the refrigerator and then assemble for lunch, reheating the burger patty in the microwave.

FOR THE RED ONION QUICK PICKLE

½ cup apple cider vinegar

½ teaspoon sea salt

½ teaspoon honey

½ red onion, very thinly sliced

FOR THE GARLIC MAYO

6 tablespoons olive oil mayonnaise

3 garlic cloves, finely minced

Pinch sea salt

TO MAKE THE RED ONION QUICK PICKLE

1. In a medium bowl, whisk together the vinegar, salt, and honey.
2. Add the red onions. Cover and allow to sit for 30 minutes or while burgers cook.

TO MAKE THE GARLIC MAYO

In a small bowl, whisk together the mayonnaise, garlic, and sea salt. Refrigerate, covered, until you're ready to use it.

FOR THE BURGERS

¾ pound ground beef

¾ pound bulk Italian sausage

3 garlic cloves, minced

1 large egg, beaten

¼ cup bread crumbs

1 tablespoon dried
Italian herbs

Pinch red pepper flakes

½ teaspoon sea salt

6 whole-wheat hamburger
buns, toasted

TO MAKE THE BURGERS

1. Preheat your oven to 375°F. Place a wire rack over a rimmed baking sheet.

2. In a large bowl, combine the ground beef, Italian sausage, garlic, eggs, bread crumbs, Italian herbs, red pepper flakes, and sea salt.

3. Mix well and form into 6 patties. Place the patties on the prepared baking sheet.

4. Bake until the patties reach an internal temperature of 165°F, about 20 minutes.

5. To assemble the burgers, spread 2 tablespoons of the mayonnaise on the buns. Top each with a patty and the pickled onion slices.

. . . .

SUBSTITUTION TIP: If you prefer a spicier burger, you can use hot Italian sausage. You can also add additional veggie fixings to these burgers such as sliced tomatoes or shredded lettuce.

. . . .

PER SERVING: Calories: 519; Total fat: 33g; Saturated fat: 13g; Carbohydrates: 30g; Fiber: 5g; Protein: 26g

Asian Pork Tenderloin with Spicy Red Cabbage Slaw

SERVES 6 / PREP TIME: 15 MINUTES, PLUS 8 HOURS TO MARINATE / COOK TIME: 30 MINUTES

Get the pork marinating before you head out in the morning, and you can pop this in the oven when you get home and prepare the slaw while the pork cooks. You can even mix up the marinade the night before and then simply pour it into a zip-top bag with the pork in the morning.

FOR THE PORK

¼ cup low-sodium soy sauce (or tamari for gluten-free)

1 tablespoon freshly grated ginger

1 Asian pear, peeled, with core and seeds removed, roughly chopped

2 tablespoons sesame oil

1 teaspoon sriracha

2 tablespoons pure maple syrup

4 green onions, minced

4 garlic cloves, minced

1½ pounds pork tenderloin

TO MAKE THE PORK

1. In a blender or food processor, combine the soy sauce, ginger, Asian pear, sesame oil, sriracha, maple syrup, green onions, and garlic. Pulse for 20 one-second pulses, or until smooth.

2. Pour into a zip-top bag with the tenderloin, making sure the marinade coats the meat. Refrigerate for 8 hours.

3. Preheat your oven to 450°F. Remove the pork from the marinade and pat it dry with paper towels.

4. Place on a roasting rack in a roasting pan and cook in the preheated oven for 25 minutes, or until the internal temperature of the pork is 145°F. Remove from the oven and rest for 5 minutes before slicing.

FOR THE SLAW

1 head red cabbage, shredded

1 bunch green onions, thinly sliced

¼ cup chopped fresh cilantro

2 tablespoons apple cider vinegar

3 tablespoons extra-virgin olive oil

3 garlic cloves, minced

1 teaspoon freshly grated ginger

1 teaspoon Chinese hot mustard

¼ teaspoon sea salt

TO MAKE THE SLAW

1. In a large bowl, combine the cabbage, green onions, and cilantro.
2. In a small bowl, whisk together the apple cider vinegar, olive oil, garlic, ginger, mustard, and salt. Pour over the cabbage and toss to mix.
3. Serve as a side with the pork tenderloin.

. . . .

COOKING TIP: A quick way to shred the cabbage is to grate it on a box grater. You can also use the shredding attachment to a food processor.

. . . .

PER SERVING: Calories: 320; Total fat: 17g; Saturated fat: 4g; Carbohydrates: 22g; Fiber: 5g; Protein: 22g

Balsamic-Glazed Pork Tenderloin

LEFTOVERS LUNCH SERVES 6 / PREP TIME: 15 MINUTES / COOK TIME: 35 MINUTES

You can use leftovers in a lunch salad or as a sandwich filling, or simply enjoy leftovers the next day along with some fresh veggies. The balsamic glaze adds sweetness to the earthy pork. If you like a bit of heat, add a pinch of red pepper flakes to the balsamic glaze.

2 tablespoons extra-virgin olive oil

1½ pounds pork tenderloin

½ teaspoon sea salt

¼ teaspoon freshly cracked black pepper

½ cup balsamic vinegar

Juice of 1 orange

2 tablespoons honey or pure maple syrup

1 garlic clove, minced

2 tablespoons minced shallot

½ teaspoon dried sage

1. Preheat your oven to 450°F. Place a roasting rack in a roasting pan.
2. In a large skillet, heat the olive oil on medium-high until it shimmers.
3. Season the tenderloin with the salt and pepper and sear it in the skillet until browned on all sides, about 4 minutes per side.
4. Remove the pork from the skillet and place it on the prepared roasting rack.
5. Add the vinegar, orange juice, honey, garlic, shallot, and sage to the skillet, scraping any browned bits from the bottom of the pan with the side of a spoon.
6. Bring to a simmer and simmer until the liquid is reduced by half, about 5 minutes.
7. Brush the glaze onto the pork, reserving any leftover glaze in the pan.
8. Roast the pork in the preheated oven until the internal temperature of the pork is 145°F, 20 to 25 minutes. Remove from the oven and rest for 5 minutes before slicing.
9. While the pork rests, bring any remaining glaze to a boil on the stove. Pour over the pork.

ON THE MENU: Make a complete meal by serving this with the Spinach and Strawberry Salad on page 72.

PER SERVING: Calories: 210; Total fat: 10g; Saturated fat: 3g; Carbohydrates: 11g; Fiber: <1g; Protein: 19g

Pork Chops with Apples and Cabbage

ONE POT, LEFTOVERS LUNCH

SERVES 6 / PREP TIME: 10 MINUTES / COOK TIME: 20 MINUTES

Apple, pork, and cabbage is a classic flavor combination that makes a delicious and hearty meal. The sweetness of the apples pairs beautifully with the savory pork and earthy cabbage. The one-inch-thick boneless pork chops cook quickly on the stovetop, so this is a relatively fast meal.

2 tablespoons extra-virgin olive oil

6 thin-cut pork chops

1 teaspoon sea salt, divided

¼ teaspoon freshly cracked black pepper

2 tablespoons fresh rosemary, finely chopped

3 tablespoons apple cider vinegar

½ cup low-sodium chicken or vegetable broth

3 cups shredded red cabbage

2 sweet-tart apples, peeled, cored, and sliced

1. In a large skillet, heat the olive oil on medium-high until it shimmers.
2. Season the pork chops with ½ teaspoon of salt, the pepper, and the rosemary.
3. Add to the skillet and cook until browned on each side and cooked through, 4 to 5 minutes per side.
4. Set the pork aside on a platter tented with foil to keep warm.
5. Return the pan to the heat. Add the vinegar and broth, using the side of the spoon to scrape any browned bits from the bottom of the pan.
6. Add the cabbage and apples. Season with the remaining ½ teaspoon of salt. Cook, stirring occasionally, until the vegetables are tender, about 6 minutes.
7. Serve the pork on top of the apples and cabbage or spoon the apples and cabbage over the pork chops.

SUBSTITUTION TIP: You can save time by using coleslaw mix in place of the cabbage. You'll find coleslaw mix with the bagged salads in the produce section of the grocery store.

PER SERVING: Calories: 216; Total fat: 10g; Saturated fat: 3g; Carbohydrates: 9g; Fiber: 2g; Protein: 22g

Greek-Style Pork Chops with Olive Salsa

LEFTOVERS LUNCH

SERVES 6 / PREP TIME: 10 MINUTES, PLUS 8 HOURS TO MARINATE / COOK TIME: 10 MINUTES

. . . .

Marinating these pork chops makes them flavorful and juicy. Meanwhile, the olive salsa adds fresh flavors that perfectly complement the earthy flavors of the pork. You can make the salsa up to 8 hours ahead of time and refrigerate it to allow the flavors to blend.

. . . .

4 tablespoons extra-virgin olive oil, divided

Juice of 2 lemons

2 teaspoons oregano

1 tablespoon Dijon mustard

1 teaspoon sea salt, divided

¼ teaspoon black pepper

1 teaspoon garlic powder

1 teaspoon onion powder

6 boneless thin-cut pork chops

½ cup Spanish olives, pitted and chopped

½ cup chopped black olives

Zest of 1 lemon

½ red onion, minced

2 large tomatoes, chopped

3 garlic cloves, minced

1 tablespoon apple cider vinegar

Pinch red pepper flakes

1. In a small bowl, whisk together 2 tablespoons of olive oil with the lemon juice, oregano, mustard, ½ teaspoon of sea salt, black pepper, garlic powder, and onion powder.
2. Place the pork chops in a large zip-top bag and pour the marinade over the top, taking care to coat the chops. Seal and marinate in the refrigerator for 8 hours.
3. In a large skillet, heat the remaining 2 tablespoons of olive oil on medium-high until it shimmers. Remove the chops from the marinade and pat them dry with a paper towel. Cook in the hot oil until browned, 4 to 5 minutes per side.
4. Meanwhile, combine the olives, lemon zest, red onion, tomatoes, garlic, apple cider vinegar, red pepper flakes, and remaining ½ teaspoon of sea salt in a medium bowl. Stir to combine.
5. Serve the chops with the salsa spooned over the top.

. . . .

THE GOOD STUFF: Olives and olive oil are both rich in oleocanthal, which can help alleviate symptoms of osteoarthritis.

. . . .

PER SERVING: Calories: 274; Total fat: 17g; Saturated fat: 4g; Carbohydrates: 7g; Fiber: 1g; Protein: 22g

Canadian Bacon and Veggie Pita Pizzas

QUICK & EASY SERVES 4 / PREP TIME: 10 MINUTES / COOK TIME: 10 MINUTES

The great thing about pita pizza—besides how quick and easy it is to make—is that you can top it with anything you like. Feel free to experiment with your own favorite toppings. This version uses Canadian bacon, artichoke hearts, red onion, and olives to make a tasty, OA-friendly meal or snack.

2 tablespoons extra-virgin olive oil

2 tablespoons minced shallots

3 garlic cloves, minced

1 (14-ounce) can crushed tomatoes and basil, undrained

1 tablespoon dried Italian herbs

4 whole-wheat pitas

8 ounces Canadian bacon or ham, chopped

½ cup canned artichoke hearts, drained and chopped

½ red onion, finely diced

½ cup chopped black olives

1 cup shredded part-skim mozzarella cheese

1. Preheat your oven to 400°F.
2. In a small pot, heat the olive oil on medium-high until it shimmers. Add the shallots and cook, stirring occasionally, until soft, about 3 minutes. Add the garlic and cook, stirring constantly, for 30 seconds.
3. Add the crushed tomatoes and Italian herbs. Bring to a simmer. Simmer, stirring, until the sauce thickens, about 4 minutes.
4. Place the pita rounds on a rimmed baking sheet. Spread each with the tomato sauce. Top with the Canadian bacon, artichoke hearts, red onion, and black olives. Sprinkle the cheese over the top.
5. Bake in the preheated oven until the cheese is melted and starting to brown, about 10 minutes.

SUBSTITUTION TIP: Save time by using a premade bottled spaghetti sauce in place of the canned tomatoes, garlic, shallots, and Italian herbs.

PER SERVING: Calories: 453; Total fat: 20g; Saturated fat: 6g; Carbohydrates: 43g; Fiber: 8g; Protein: 29g

Lamb Chili

ONE POT, LEFTOVERS LUNCH **SERVES 6 / PREP TIME: 10 MINUTES / COOK TIME: 20 MINUTES**

Lamb brings an interesting, hearty flavor to chili. This chili keeps very well in the refrigerator for up to a week or in the freezer for up to six months. You can even put the chili ingredients (with the browned ground lamb) in the slow cooker and cook it on low for 8 hours.

1 pound ground lamb

1 white onion, chopped

1 red bell pepper, seeds and ribs removed, chopped

2 (14-ounce) cans low-sodium kidney beans, drained

2 (14-ounce) cans crushed tomatoes, undrained

½ cup water

2 tablespoons chili powder

1 teaspoon garlic powder

1 teaspoon dried oregano

½ teaspoon ground cumin

½ teaspoon sea salt

½ red onion, minced

¼ cup chopped fresh cilantro

½ cup shredded Monterey Jack cheese

1. In a large pot, cook the ground lamb on medium-high, crumbling as you cook, until the lamb is browned, about 5 minutes.
2. Add the white onion and red bell pepper and cook, stirring occasionally, until the veggies are soft, about 4 minutes.
3. Add the kidney beans, crushed tomatoes, water, chili powder, garlic powder, oregano, cumin, and salt. Bring to a simmer. Cook, stirring occasionally, for 10 minutes.
4. Serve with the red onion, cilantro, and cheese as garnish.

SUBSTITUTION TIP: You can also use ground beef or ground pork in place of the lamb in this recipe.

PER SERVING: Calories: 394; Total fat: 14g; Saturated fat: 8g; Carbohydrates: 42g; Fiber: 10g; Protein: 25g

Lamb Meatballs with Lemon Kale

LEFTOVERS LUNCH SERVES 8 / PREP TIME: 10 MINUTES / COOK TIME: 20 MINUTES

These meatballs freeze really well. Freeze them in zip-top bags in single servings for lunch. The kale is best eaten right after it's prepared, so when taking the meatballs for a leftovers lunch, plan to have a side dish with them such as a salad or some quick steamed veggies.

2 pounds ground lamb

1 red onion, grated

6 garlic cloves, minced

1 teaspoon ground cumin

1 teaspoon dried oregano

1 teaspoon ground coriander

Zest of 1 lemon

1 teaspoon sea salt, divided

¼ teaspoon freshly cracked black pepper

2 tablespoons extra-virgin olive oil

4 cups kale, stems removed, chopped

Juice of 1 lemon

1. Preheat your oven to 425°F.
2. In a large bowl, combine the lamb, red onion, garlic, cumin, oregano, coriander, lemon zest, ½ teaspoon of sea salt, and the pepper. Roll into meatballs that are about 2 tablespoons and place them in a single layer on a rimmed baking sheet. Bake in the preheated oven until the lamb reaches an internal temperature of 160°F, about 20 minutes.
3. While the lamb cooks, heat the olive oil on medium-high in a large skillet until it shimmers.
4. Add the kale and season with the remaining ½ teaspoon of salt. Cook, stirring occasionally, for 4 minutes. Add the lemon juice. Cook, stirring occasionally, until the juice reduces, about 5 minutes more.

THE GOOD STUFF: Kale is especially high in quercetin and sulforaphane, a flavonoid and an antioxidant, respectively, that are beneficial for people with OA.

PER SERVING: Calories: 374; Total fat: 27g; Saturated fat: 13g; Carbohydrates: 11g; Fiber: 2g; Protein: 25g

Ground Beef Kofta with Veggie Couscous

LEFTOVERS LUNCH **SERVES 6 / PREP TIME: 10 MINUTES / COOK TIME: 20 MINUTES**

. . . .

You don't need to use skewers to make these kofta, but if you enjoy your meat on sticks, then you're certainly welcome to do so. Otherwise, just shape the kofta into sausage shapes and bake them without the sticks. If you do use wooden skewers, then you'll need to soak them for about 20 minutes before baking.

. . . .

FOR THE KOFTA

1½ pounds ground beef

½ red onion, grated, with the water squeezed out

4 garlic cloves, minced

¼ cup finely chopped fresh Italian parsley

1 teaspoon ground cumin

1 teaspoon ground coriander

½ teaspoon sea salt

¼ teaspoon freshly cracked black pepper

FOR THE COUSCOUS

2 tablespoons extra-virgin olive oil

½ red onion, chopped

1 carrot, peeled and chopped

1 red bell pepper, seeds and ribs removed, chopped

1½ cups unsalted chicken broth

½ teaspoon sea salt

1½ cups instant couscous

TO MAKE THE KOFTA

1. Preheat your oven to 425°F.
2. In a large bowl, combine the ground beef, red onion, garlic, parsley, cumin, coriander, salt, and pepper.
3. Divide the meat into 12 even pieces and roll into oblong shapes. If using skewers, mold them around the skewers.
4. Place the kofta on a rimmed baking sheet and bake in the preheated oven until the meat reaches an internal temperature of 160°F, about 20 minutes.

TO MAKE THE COUSCOUS

1. While the beef cooks, in a medium saucepan, heat the olive oil on medium-high until it shimmers.
2. Add the onion, carrot, and bell pepper and cook, stirring, until the veggies soften, about 5 minutes.
3. Add the chicken broth and salt and bring it to a simmer.
4. Add the couscous. Stir. Remove from the heat, cover, and let it sit for 10 minutes. Fluff with a fork before serving.

. . . .

COOKING TIP: To squeeze the water out of the onion, roll the grated onion in a tea towel and wring it over the sink.

. . . .

PER SERVING: Calories: 406; Total fat: 16g; Saturated fat: 5g; Carbohydrates: 38g; Fiber: 3g; Protein: 29g

Flank Steak with Romesco Sauce

LEFTOVERS LUNCH **SERVES 8 / PREP TIME: 10 MINUTES / COOK TIME: 25 MINUTES**

Romesco sauce is a quick and easy puréed red pepper sauce that's delicious on steak. If you like it, you can also try it on vegetables, fish, or poultry. This version is very simple—it takes about five minutes to prepare, and it will keep in the refrigerator for up to a week.

FOR THE FLANK STEAK

½ teaspoon sea salt

¼ teaspoon freshly cracked black pepper

1 teaspoon garlic powder

1 teaspoon brown sugar

1 teaspoon dried thyme

1 (2-pound) flank steak

FOR THE ROMESCO SAUCE

1 (12-ounce) jar roasted red peppers, drained

Juice of one lemon

5 cherry tomatoes, halved

½ cup almonds

¼ cup fresh Italian parsley

3 garlic cloves, minced

2 tablespoons extra-virgin olive oil

TO MAKE THE FLANK STEAK

1. In a small bowl, mix the salt, pepper, garlic powder, brown sugar, and thyme.
2. Rub on the steak.
3. Heat a grill pan on medium-high.
4. Add the steak to the hot pan. Cook until the steak reaches an internal temperature of 135°F, about 8 minutes per side.
5. Allow to rest, tented with foil, for 10 minutes.
6. Slice the steak.

TO MAKE THE ROMESCO SAUCE

Combine all ingredients in a blender or food processor and blend until smooth. Top the sliced steak with sauce to serve.

COOKING TIP: The trick to tender flank steak is cutting it on the bias. After allowing the steak to rest for about 10 minutes after cooking, locate the grain of the steak and cut against the grain to shorten the fibers and make the steak more tender.

PER SERVING: Calories: 270; Total fat: 15g; Saturated fat: 1g; Carbohydrates: 6g; Fiber: 2g; Protein: 27g

Beef and Asparagus Stir-Fry

QUICK & EASY, ONE POT, LEFTOVERS LUNCH

SERVES 6 / PREP TIME: 10 MINUTES / COOK TIME: 20 MINUTES

Stir-fries make great weeknight meals because they come together so quickly. They're even quicker and easier if you pick up pre-cut veggies to save prep time. While this stir-fry calls for beef, asparagus, bell peppers, and mushrooms, you can substitute your favorite veggies as well.

2 tablespoons extra-virgin olive oil

1½ pounds beef sirloin, cut into ½-inch-thick strips

1 red onion, sliced

1 red bell pepper, seeds and ribs removed, sliced

1 bunch asparagus, woody ends removed, chopped

8 ounces shiitake mushrooms, sliced

3 garlic cloves, minced

2 tablespoons low-sodium soy sauce

¼ cup low-sodium chicken broth

½ teaspoon sriracha

1 tablespoon freshly grated ginger

1 teaspoon cornstarch

1. In a large skillet or wok, heat the olive oil on medium-high until it shimmers.
2. Add the beef and cook, stirring, until browned, about 5 minutes. Remove the beef from the fat in the pan with a slotted spoon and set it aside.
3. In the same pan, add the onion, bell pepper, asparagus, and mushrooms. Cook, stirring occasionally, until the veggies soften and begin to brown, 5 to 7 minutes. Add the garlic and cook, stirring constantly, for 30 seconds. Return the beef to the pan.
4. In a small bowl, whisk together the soy sauce, chicken broth, sriracha, ginger, and cornstarch.
5. Add to the pan with the beef and veggies. Cook, stirring, until the sauce thickens, about 3 minutes more.

ON THE MENU: Serve this with a side of steamed brown rice or rice noodles for a delicious meal.

PER SERVING: Calories: 328; Total fat: 14g; Saturated fat: 4g; Carbohydrates: 13g; Fiber: 3g; Protein: 38g

Beef Fajitas with Guacamole

QUICK & EASY, LEFTOVERS LUNCH

SERVES 6 / PREP TIME: 10 MINUTES, PLUS 8 HOURS TO MARINATE / COOK TIME: 20 MINUTES

. . . .

Beef can marinate in the refrigerator for quite a while. In fact, if you like, you can marinate the beef overnight and cook it when you get home the next evening. For this recipe, you'll set aside about 1 tablespoon of marinade to mix with the cooked meat for additional flavor.

. . . .

4 tablespoons extra-virgin olive oil, divided

1 bunch green onions, chopped

1 jalapeño pepper, stems and seeds removed, chopped

½ cup fresh cilantro leaves, divided

¾ teaspoon sea salt, divided

Juice of 3 limes, divided

4 garlic cloves, minced

1½ pounds flank steak

6 whole-wheat tortillas

1 green bell pepper, seeds and ribs removed, sliced

1 white onion, sliced

2 avocados, peeled, pitted, and cubed

¼ red onion, finely chopped

1. In a blender or food processor, combine 2 tablespoons of olive oil, the green onions, the jalapeño, ¼ cup of cilantro, ½ teaspoon of salt, the juice of 2 limes, and the garlic. Pulse for 20 one-second pulses or until it makes a paste. Set aside 1 tablespoon of the marinade in a small bowl in the refrigerator.

2. Place the flank steak in a zip-top bag and add the remaining marinade, making sure the beef is coated. Seal and refrigerate for at least 8 hours.

3. Preheat your oven to 300°F. Wrap the tortillas in foil and place in the oven to warm for 10 minutes.

4. Remove the meat from the marinade and use a paper towel to wipe away any excess.

5. In a large skillet, heat the remaining 2 tablespoons of olive oil on medium-high until it shimmers. Add the beef and cook until it reaches an internal temperature of 135°F, about 6 minutes per side. Remove the beef from the pan and set it aside, tented with foil to keep warm.

6. Return the pan to the heat. Add the green bell pepper and sliced onion and cook, stirring occasionally, until the vegetables are soft, about 5 minutes.

7. Slice the beef on the bias into ½-inch thick slices and return it to the pan with the vegetables. Add the reserved marinade to the pan. Cook, stirring, for 1 minute.

CONTINUED ▸

8. In a medium bowl, combine the avocado, the remaining ¼ cup of cilantro, the juice of 1 lime, the remaining ¼ teaspoon of sea salt, and the chopped red onion. Mash with a fork to mix.

9. Serve the beef and veggies with the tortillas topped with the guacamole.

ON THE MENU: If you like, you can also serve this with 2 tablespoons each of nonfat Greek yogurt as a garnish similar to sour cream.

PER SERVING: Calories: 506; Total fat: 28g; Saturated fat: 4g; Carbohydrates: 33g; Fiber: 9g; Protein: 30g

Garlic Steak with Warm Spinach Salad

QUICK & EASY

SERVES 4 / PREP TIME: 10 MINUTES, PLUS 8 HOURS TO MARINATE / COOK TIME: 20 MINUTES

This garlic marinade adds tons of flavor to sirloin steaks before you cook them. While this recipe calls for a grill pan, you can also use an outdoor grill or a Foreman grill to cook the steaks. If you don't have Worcestershire sauce, you can substitute with an equal amount of low-sodium soy sauce or tamari.

½ cup balsamic vinegar

2 tablespoons Worcestershire sauce

2 tablespoons honey, divided

1 teaspoon Dijon mustard

10 garlic cloves, minced

2 tablespoons extra-virgin olive oil

4 (5-ounce) sirloin steaks

4 slices bacon

¼ cup red wine vinegar

2 tablespoons minced shallots

¼ teaspoon freshly cracked black pepper

6 cups baby spinach

1. In a small bowl, whisk together the balsamic vinegar, the Worcestershire sauce, 1 tablespoon of honey, the mustard, the garlic, and the olive oil.

2. Place the steaks in a zip-top bag and add the marinade, making sure to coat the steak. Seal and refrigerate for at least 8 hours.

3. Heat a grill pan on medium-high. Remove the steak from the marinade and pat it dry with a paper towel. Cook the steaks in the grill pan until they reach an internal temperature of 130°F, about 6 minutes per side.

4. While the steak cooks, in a large skillet, cook the bacon on medium-high heat until crisp, about 3 minutes per side.

5. Remove the bacon from the fat in the skillet and set it aside.

6. Add the red wine vinegar, shallots, remaining 1 tablespoon of honey, and pepper. Bring to a simmer and cook for 3 minutes, whisking occasionally.

7. Put the spinach in a large bowl. Pour the hot vinegar mixture over the top and crumble the bacon over the salad.

8. Slice the steak and place it atop the salad to serve.

COOKING TIP: Allow the steak to rest for about 10 minutes before serving it to allow the juices to distribute evenly through the steak.

PER SERVING: Calories: 450; Total fat: 19g; Saturated fat: 5g; Carbohydrates: 20g; Fiber: 2g; Protein: 50g

Ground Beef–Stuffed Bell Peppers

LEFTOVERS LUNCH **SERVES 6 / PREP TIME: 20 MINUTES / COOK TIME: 35 MINUTES**

Stuffed bell peppers with ground beef are a classic comfort food. You can store the leftover peppers in a zip-top bag in the refrigerator for up to three days or in the freezer for up to six months. Reheat thawed peppers for lunch in the microwave for 1 to 2 minutes depending on your microwave's power.

6 red bell peppers

1½ pounds ground beef

1 red onion, finely chopped

3 garlic cloves, minced

1 teaspoon dried thyme

2 (14-ounce) cans diced tomatoes, drained

¾ cup cooked brown rice

½ cup grated Parmesan cheese

1. Preheat your oven to 475°F.
2. Cut the tops off the peppers and carefully scoop out any seeds and ribs. Arrange the peppers, cut-side up, in a 9-by-13-inch baking pan.
3. In a skillet, cook the ground beef on medium-high, crumbling as you cook, until it is browned, about 5 minutes.
4. Add the onion and cook, stirring occasionally, until the onion is soft, about 3 minutes more.
5. Add the garlic and cook, stirring constantly, for 30 seconds.
6. Add the thyme, tomatoes, and brown rice and cook, stirring, until warmed through, about 3 minutes more.
7. Spoon the beef mixture into the peppers. Sprinkle the cheese over the top.
8. Bake in the preheated oven until the peppers are soft, about 20 minutes.

SUBSTITUTION TIP: You can also use this beef mixture to stuff small halved eggplants with some of the flesh scooped out. Baking time will increase to about 35 minutes.

PER SERVING: Calories: 326; Total fat: 13g; Saturated fat: 6g; Carbohydrates: 23g; Fiber: 4g; Protein: 30g

Beef Pinwheels with Spinach, Feta, and Pine Nuts

LEFTOVERS LUNCH

SERVES 6 / PREP TIME: 10 MINUTES, PLUS 8 HOURS TO MARINATE / COOK TIME: 35 MINUTES, PLUS 10 MINUTES TO REST

To make these pinwheels, you'll need to learn how to butterfly flank steak. To do this, cut a vertical slit lengthwise in the top of the steak until the knife goes halfway to the bottom. Then, use a sharp knife to cut into each side of the slit horizontally until you're about half an inch away from the sides of the steak. Unfold the steak like a book and pound it with a mallet to even out the depth of the steak so it cooks evenly.

½ cup red wine vinegar

2 tablespoons extra-virgin olive oil

1 teaspoon Dijon mustard

6 garlic cloves, minced

½ teaspoon sea salt

¼ teaspoon freshly cracked black pepper

1½ pounds flank steak, butterflied

1 (10-ounce) package frozen spinach, thawed, extra water squeezed out

½ cup crumbled feta

½ cup pine nuts

1. In a small bowl, whisk together the vinegar, olive oil, mustard, garlic, salt, and pepper.
2. Put the butterflied steak in a large zip-top bag and add the marinade, making sure to coat the entire steak. Refrigerate for at least 8 hours.
3. Preheat your oven to 425°F.
4. Remove the steak from the bag and pat it dry with paper towels.
5. Place the steak on a clean surface and spread the spinach in an even layer over the top of the steak. Sprinkle with the feta and pine nuts.
6. Roll into a tight roll and tie in several places with butcher's twine. Place on a rimmed baking sheet.
7. Bake in the preheated oven until the internal temperature of the steak reaches 130°F, about 35 minutes.
8. Allow to rest for 10 minutes before slicing into 6 pieces.

ON THE MENU: Serve this with baked sweet potatoes topped with ¼ cup of light sour cream or nonfat Greek yogurt.

PER SERVING: Calories: 335; Total fat: 22g; Saturated fat: 3g; Carbohydrates: 5g; Fiber: 2g; Protein: 29g

Chocolate Mousse with Raspberries, page 145

CHAPTER 9

Desserts

Honey Green Tea Sorbet

QUICK & EASY

SERVES 4 / PREP TIME: 5 MINUTES / COOK TIME: 5 MINUTES, PLUS 4 HOURS TO FREEZE

While the active time to make this sorbet is only 10 minutes, you will need to be around to stir the mixture every 30 minutes as it freezes. If you don't have that kind of time, you can also just freeze it in ice pop molds. You'll still get the flavor and benefits of green tea, but you won't need to stick around to stir it.

1 tablespoon matcha powder

½ cup honey

2 cups water

Juice and zest of 1 lemon

1. In a medium saucepan, combine the matcha, honey, water, and lemon zest.
2. Heat on medium-high, stirring, until the honey dissolves.
3. Squeeze in the lemon juice and stir.
4. Pour into a large, freezer-proof container and freeze. Stir every 30 minutes until frozen, about 4 hours.

THE GOOD STUFF: Matcha powder is made with green tea, which is an excellent source of EGCG, a polyphenol found to slow the symptoms of OA.

PER SERVING: Calories: 137; Total fat: 0g; Saturated fat: 0g; Carbohydrates: 36g; Fiber: <1g; Protein: <1g

Tart Cherry, Lime, and Coconut Freezer Pops

QUICK & EASY **SERVES 4 / PREP TIME: 5 MINUTES, PLUS 5 HOURS TO FREEZE**

You can find tart cherry juice in natural food stores, health food stores, or online. Be sure you use tart cherry juice, not regular cherry juice. Tart cherry juice has been shown to help relieve the pain of osteoarthritis, making these freezer pops a refreshing way to enjoy something sweet while doing something good for your body.

2 cups tart cherry juice

Juice of 2 limes and zest of 1 lime

2 tablespoons honey

½ cup light coconut milk

1. In a medium saucepan, combine the tart cherry juice, lime zest, and honey.
2. Heat on medium-high, stirring, until the honey dissolves.
3. Squeeze in the lime juice and add the coconut milk. Stir.
4. Pour into 4 ice pop molds and freeze until solid, around 5 hours.

COOKING TIP: If you don't have ice pop molds, don't worry. You can also pour the mixture into paper cups. Place a piece of foil over the top of each cup and insert an ice pop stick through the foil, which will hold it in place as it freezes.

PER SERVING: Calories: 127; Total fat: 2g; Saturated fat: 2g; Carbohydrates: 27g; Fiber: <1g; Protein: <1g

Pears Poached in Red Wine with Hazelnuts

ONE POT **SERVES 4 / PREP TIME: 5 MINUTES / COOK TIME: 50 MINUTES**

Pears poached in red wine is a classic, elegant dessert. This recipe brings in spicy flavors and honey to add to the delicious flavors of the wine and then finishes with crunchy hazelnuts for texture. Choose ripe but firm fruit and a dry red wine such as cabernet sauvignon for the perfect poached pear.

2 cups dry red wine

Juice of 1 orange and zest of half an orange

1 cinnamon stick

2 cardamom pods

4 cloves

½ cup honey

4 Bosc pears, peeled

¼ cup chopped hazelnuts

1. In a large saucepan, bring the wine, orange juice, orange zest, cinnamon stick, cardamom pods, cloves, and honey to a simmer on medium-high heat.

2. Add the pears. Reduce the heat to medium-low. Cover and simmer, turning the pears every 5 minutes or so until the pears are soft, about 40 minutes.

3. Remove the pan from the heat. Set the pears upright in the poaching liquid and allow it to cool on the countertop.

4. Place the pears on dessert plates and return the poaching liquid to the stove. Bring to a boil on medium-high heat and cook until the liquid reduces to a syrup, about 5 minutes.

5. Spoon over the pears and sprinkle with the hazelnuts.

SUBSTITUTION TIP: If you're not a fan of red wine, you can also use white wine or juice such as pear juice. If using juice, reduce the honey to ¼ cup.

PER SERVING: Calories: 380; Total fat: 5g; Saturated fat: <1g; Carbohydrates: 67g; Fiber: 6g; Protein: 2g

Frozen Yogurt with Mixed Berry Sauce

QUICK & EASY, ONE POT SERVES 4 / PREP TIME: 5 MINUTES / COOK TIME: 10 MINUTES

You can choose your favorite flavor of frozen yogurt for this recipe. While the recipe calls for vanilla, it's also delicious with chocolate or, if you're feeling adventurous, orange sherbet. You can use fresh or frozen berries here depending on what's in season and what's most convenient.

½ pint raspberries

½ pint blueberries

½ pint blackberries

½ pint strawberries, hulled and sliced

½ cup honey

Juice of 1 lemon

2 cups frozen vanilla yogurt

1. In a large saucepan, combine the fruit, honey, and lemon juice. Bring to a simmer over medium heat. Cook, stirring occasionally, until the berries release their liquid and become syrupy.
2. Remove from the heat and cool slightly.
3. Transfer the warm berries to a blender. Blend until smooth.
4. Serve spooned over the yogurt.

THE GOOD STUFF: All the bright red berries are full of anthocyanins, which can reduce the inflammation associated with OA.

PER SERVING: Calories: 288; Total fat: 3g; Saturated fat: 1g; Carbohydrates: 69g; Fiber: 6g; Protein: 4g

Maple-Glazed Baked Apples

ONE POT **SERVES 4 / PREP TIME: 10 MINUTES / COOK TIME: 35 MINUTES**

The best apples for this dessert are sweet-tart apples such as Cripps Pink, Honeycrisp, Braeburn, or Granny Smith. These apples are quite delicious warm straight from the oven. However, they are also tasty served chilled, so you can take them with you for a sweet snack at work or on the go.

4 medium sweet-tart apples

1 teaspoon ground cinnamon

6 tablespoons finely chopped pecans

1 tablespoon butter, chopped into small pieces

¼ cup pure maple syrup

1. Preheat your oven to 375°F.
2. Slice the tops off the apples and use a spoon or sharp knife to remove the core, keeping the bottom part of the apple intact to serve as a bowl for the filling.
3. Place the apples in a 9-inch baking pan.
4. In a small bowl, combine the cinnamon, pecans, and butter.
5. Spoon the mixture into the cavities of the apples.
6. Drizzle the syrup over the top.
7. Bake in the preheated oven until the apples are soft, about 35 minutes.

ON THE MENU: While these are delicious alone, try serving them with a small scoop of vanilla frozen yogurt on the side.

PER SERVING: Calories: 227; Total fat: 11g; Saturated fat: 3g; Carbohydrates: 34g; Fiber: 5g; Protein: 1g

Maple Pudding with Warm Peach Compote

QUICK & EASY SERVES 6 / PREP TIME: 10 MINUTES / COOK TIME: 15 MINUTES

Use fresh or frozen peaches for this recipe, but not canned. If you're using frozen peaches, make sure that they haven't been frozen in a sugar syrup. Pudding is super easy to make homemade, but you can also purchase sugar-free vanilla pudding from the grocery store to save time.

FOR THE PUDDING

2½ cups skim milk or nondairy milk, divided

3 tablespoons cornstarch

¾ cup pure maple syrup

½ teaspoon pure vanilla extract

1 tablespoon unsalted butter

Pinch salt

FOR THE PEACHES

2 tablespoons unsalted butter

4 peaches, peeled, pitted, and sliced

1 teaspoon ground cinnamon

¼ cup pure maple syrup

TO MAKE THE PUDDING

1. In a small bowl, whisk together 1 cup of milk and the cornstarch. Set aside.
2. In a medium saucepan, heat the remaining 1½ cups of milk and the syrup on medium-high, stirring constantly. Bring to a rolling boil.
3. Reduce the heat to medium. Whisk in the milk-and-cornstarch mixture off the heat and then return the pan to the burner. Cook, whisking constantly, until the pudding thickens, about 2 minutes.
4. Remove from the heat and whisk in the vanilla, butter, and salt.
5. Transfer to 6 dessert bowls and refrigerate to chill.

TO MAKE THE PEACHES

1. In a large skillet, melt the butter on medium-high until it bubbles.
2. Add the peaches and the cinnamon. Cook, stirring occasionally, until the peaches soften, about 5 minutes.
3. Add the syrup. Cook, stirring, until the syrup thickens slightly, about 3 minutes more.
4. Serve spooned over the pudding.

SUBSTITUTION TIP: You can also serve the peaches spooned over vanilla frozen yogurt.

PER SERVING: Calories: 268; Total fat: 6g; Saturated fat: 4g; Carbohydrates: 51g; Fiber: 2g; Protein: 4g

Spiced Applesauce with Hazelnuts

ONE POT **SERVES 6 / PREP TIME: 10 MINUTES / COOK TIME: 20 MINUTES**

The hazelnuts bring a delightful crunch to this dish. You can use more than one type of apple in this recipe to add flavor and texture, but you can also use a single variety if you prefer. Choose sweet-tart apples such as Braeburn, Granny Smith, or Honeycrisp for the best flavor.

6 apples, peeled, cored, and chopped

¾ cup water

¼ cup honey or pure maple syrup

1 tablespoon freshly grated ginger

1 teaspoon ground cinnamon

½ cup chopped hazelnuts

1. In a large pot, combine the apples, water, honey, ginger, and cinnamon.
2. Bring to a simmer on medium-high heat. Cover and cook until the apples soften, about 20 minutes.
3. Remove from heat and allow to cool.
4. Use a potato masher to mash slightly.
5. Serve sprinkled with the hazelnuts.

COOKING TIP: For a smoother applesauce, once it has cooled, purée the cooked apples in a blender or a food processor.

PER SERVING: Calories: 178; Total fat: 6g; Saturated fat: <1g; Carbohydrates: 33g; Fiber: 5g; Protein: 2g

Baked Berry Compote with Crumble Topping

SERVES 6 / PREP TIME: 15 MINUTES / COOK TIME: 45 MINUTES

Use fresh berries for this compote. While frozen berries can be more convenient, they may wind up making the final mixture too wet. Feel free to switch up the berries you use in the recipe, provided that you use 3 pints of berries total to make the filling.

Nonstick cooking spray

1 pint blueberries

1 pint blackberries

1 pint raspberries

½ cup flour, divided

½ teaspoon ground cinnamon

¼ cup honey

¾ cup rolled oats

6 tablespoons brown sugar

4 tablespoons unsalted butter

1. Preheat your oven to 350°F. Spray a 9-inch square baking pan with nonstick cooking spray.
2. In a medium bowl, combine the blueberries, the blackberries, the raspberries, ¼ cup of flour, and the cinnamon. Mix well. Stir in the honey.
3. Pour the berry mixture into the prepared baking pan.
4. In another bowl, combine the oats, remaining ¼ cup of flour, brown sugar, and butter. Using your hands, mix the ingredients, using your fingertips to rub the butter into the other ingredients. For a finer topping, you can pulse the ingredients in a food processor for 20 one-second pulses or until it resembles coarse sand.
5. Pour over the berries in an even layer.
6. Bake in the preheated oven until the topping is browned and the berries are bubbly, about 45 minutes.
7. Serve warm or chilled.

SUBSTITUTION TIP: You can make this gluten-free by using gluten-free oats and gluten-free all-purpose flour.

PER SERVING: Calories: 288; Total fat: 9g; Saturated fat: 5g; Carbohydrates: 56g; Fiber: 8g; Protein: 3g

Pistachio Meringue Cookies

SERVES 12 / PREP TIME: 10 MINUTES / COOK TIME: 40 MINUTES, PLUS 2 HOURS TO COOL

For this recipe, two cookies make one serving. They'll keep well in a tightly sealed container or zip-top bag at room temperature for up to one week. You can also freeze them for up to six months, so they're a perfect dessert to make whenever you want a sweet treat.

1 cup shelled and finely chopped pistachios

Zest of 1 orange

6 tablespoons erythritol sweetener (such as Swerve), divided

3 egg whites at room temperature

¼ teaspoon cream of tartar

1. Preheat your oven to 250°F. Line a rimmed baking sheet with parchment paper.
2. In a small bowl, combine the pistachios, orange zest, and 1 tablespoon of sweetener, mixing well.
3. Using a stand mixer or eggbeater, beat the egg whites on medium until the eggs are frothy, about 1 minute.
4. Continue beating on medium, adding the cream of tartar and 1 tablespoon of sweetener at a time until you've mixed in the remaining 5 tablespoons. Beat until stiff peaks form.
5. Carefully fold in the pistachio mixture.
6. Spoon onto the prepared cookie sheet in 24 mounds.
7. Bake in the preheated oven for 20 minutes. Reduce the heat to 200°F and continue baking until the meringues begin to brown, another 20 minutes.
8. Turn off the oven. Allow the meringues to sit in the oven as it cools for 2 hours.
9. Peel from the parchment and store in zip-top bags or an airtight container.

COOKING TIP: To make the best meringue, make sure there's not even a trace of fat in any of your ingredients or utensils. Wash and dry the bowl and beaters and make sure no egg yolks get in the whites.

PER SERVING: Calories: 61; Total fat: 4g; Saturated fat: 1g; Carbohydrates: 3g; Fiber: 1g; Protein: 3g

Chocolate Mousse with Raspberries

QUICK & EASY

SERVES 4 / PREP TIME: 10 MINUTES / COOK TIME: 5 MINUTES, PLUS 2 HOURS TO CHILL

The healthy secret behind this chocolate mousse is nonfat Greek yogurt. The yogurt makes it creamy and delicious without the additional fat and calories you'd get from heavy cream. The mousse is fast and easy to make, although you'll have to wait until it has chilled to eat it.

½ cup skim milk

1 cup chocolate chips

3 tablespoons pure maple syrup

2 cups nonfat plain Greek yogurt

¼ teaspoon vanilla extract

Pinch sea salt

1 cup fresh raspberries

1. In a small saucepan, combine the milk and chocolate chips. Cook, stirring constantly, until the chocolate chips are melted and blend with the milk. Allow to cool for 5 minutes.
2. In a mixing bowl, combine the maple syrup, Greek yogurt, vanilla, and salt. Whisk to combine.
3. Stir in the chocolate-and-milk mixture. Spoon into 4 bowls. Chill for at least 2 hours.
4. Serve topped with raspberries.

SUBSTITUTION TIP: You can substitute sugar-free chocolate chips or low-sugar dark chocolate (such as Lily's dark chocolate) that has been chopped in place of the chocolate chips.

PER SERVING: Calories: 405; Total fat: 18g; Saturated fat: 10g; Carbohydrates: 56g; Fiber: 2g; Protein: 17g

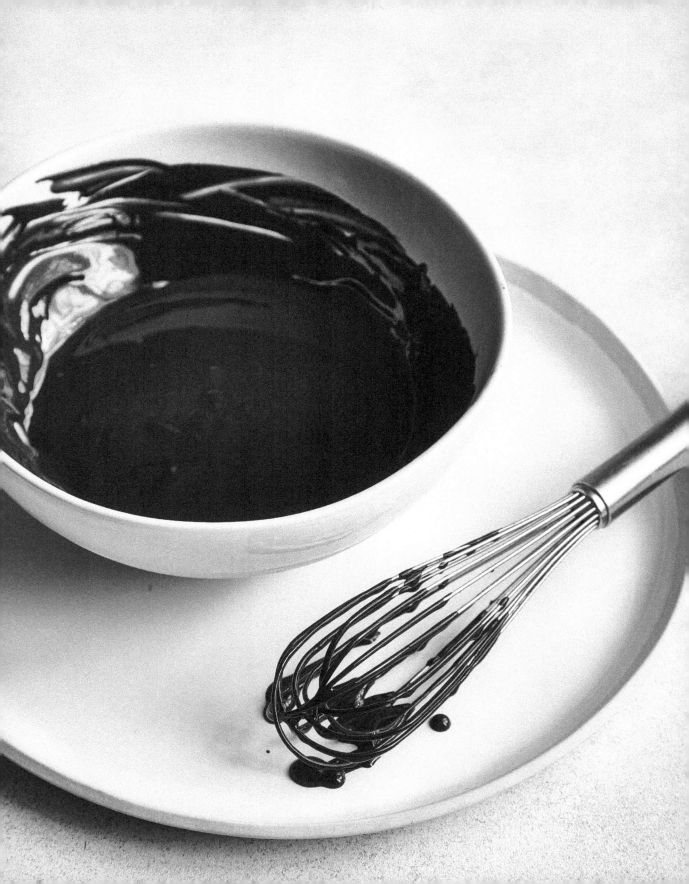

MEASUREMENT CHARTS

VOLUME EQUIVALENTS (LIQUID)

US STANDARD	US STANDARD (OUNCES)	METRIC (APPROXIMATE)
2 tablespoons	1 fl. oz.	30 mL
¼ cup	2 fl. oz.	60 mL
½ cup	4 fl. oz.	120 mL
1 cup	8 fl. oz.	240 mL
1½ cups	12 fl. oz.	355 mL
2 cups or 1 pint	16 fl. oz.	475 mL
4 cups or 1 quart	32 fl. oz.	1 L
1 gallon	128 fl. oz.	4 L

OVEN TEMPERATURES

FAHRENHEIT	CELSIUS (APPROXIMATE)
250°F	120°C
300°F	150°C
325°F	165°C
350°F	180°C
375°F	190°C
400°F	200°C
425°F	220°C
450°F	230°C

VOLUME EQUIVALENTS (DRY)

US STANDARD	METRIC (APPROXIMATE)
⅛ teaspoon	0.5 mL
¼ teaspoon	1 mL
½ teaspoon	2 mL
¾ teaspoon	4 mL
1 teaspoon	5 mL
1 tablespoon	15 mL
¼ cup	59 mL
⅓ cup	79 mL
½ cup	118 mL
⅔ cup	156 mL
¾ cup	177 mL
1 cup	235 mL
2 cups or 1 pint	475 mL
3 cups	700 mL
4 cups or 1 quart	1 L

WEIGHT EQUIVALENTS

US STANDARD	METRIC (APPROXIMATE)
½ ounce	15 g
1 ounce	30 g
2 ounces	60 g
4 ounces	115 g
8 ounces	225 g
12 ounces	340 g
16 ounces or 1 pound	455 g

REFERENCES

Arthritis by the Numbers. Accessed November 12, 2019. https://www.arthritis
.org/getmedia/e1256607-fa87-4593-aa8a-8db4f291072a/2019-ABTN-final
-March-2019.pdf

"Acetaminophen and Ibuprofen Combination Risks." Accessed November 12,
2019. https://arthritis.org/drug-guide/medication-topics/
taking-acetaminophen-safely.

"Acetaminophen Safety | Tylenol Safety." Accessed November 12, 2019.
http://www.arthritis.org/drug-guide/analgesics/analgesics.

Bannuru, Raveendhara R., Christopher H. Schmid, David M. Kent, Elizaveta E.
Vaysbrot, John B. Wong, and Timothy E. McAlindon. "Comparative Effectiveness of Pharmacologic Interventions for Knee Osteoarthritis: A Systematic
Review and Network Meta-Analysis." *Annals of Internal Medicine* 162, no. 1
(2015): 46–54.

Basu, Arpita, Jace Schell, and R. Hal Scofield. "Dietary Fruits and Arthritis."
Food & Function 9, no. 1 (January 2018): 70–7.

Beattie, Julie, Alan Crozier, and Garry G. Duthie. "Potential Health Benefits
of Berries." *Current Nutrition and Food Science* 1, no. 1 (January 2005): 71–86.

Belcaro, Gianni, Maria Rosaria Cesarone, Mark Dugall, et al. "Efficacy and
Safety of Meriva®, a Curcumin-Phosphatidylcholine Complex, During
Extended Administration in Osteoarthritis Patients." *Alternative Medicine
Review* 15, no. 4 (December 2010): 337–44.

Bello, Alfonso E., and Steffen Oesser. "Collagen Hydrolysate for the Treatment of Osteoarthritis and Other Joint Disorders: A Review of the Literature."
Current Medical Research and Opinion 22, no. 11 (November 2006): 2221–32.

Berenbaum, Francis, Florent Eymard, and Xavier Houard. "Osteoarthritis,
Inflammation, and Obesity." *Current Opinion in Rheumatology* 25, no. 1
(2013): 114–18.

Boe, Chelsea, and C. Thomas Vangsness. "Fish Oil and Osteoarthritis: Current Evidence." *American Journal of Orthopedics* 44, no. 7 (July 2015): 302–5.

Borlinghaus, Jan, Frank Albrecht, Martin C. H. Gruhlke, Ifeanyi D. Nwachukwu, and Alan Slusarenko. "Allicin: Chemistry and Biological Properties." *Molecules* 19, no. 8 (August 2014): 12591–618.

Christiansen, Blaine A., Simrit Bhatti, Ramin Goudarzi, and Shahin Emami. "Management of Osteoarthritis with Avocado/Soybean Unsaponifiables." *Cartilage* 6, no. 1 (January 2015): 30–44.

Christensen R., Elsa Marie Bartels, Arne Astrup, and Henning Bliddal. "Symptomatic Efficacy of Avocado-Soybean Unsaponifiables (ASU) in Osteoarthritis (OA) Patients: A Meta-Analysis of Randomized Controlled Trials." *Osteoarthritis and Cartilage* 16, no. 4 (2008): 399–408.

Davidson, Rose, Orla Jupp, Rachel de Ferrars, et al. "Sulforaphane Represses Matrix-Degrading Proteases and Protects Cartilage from Destruction In Vitro and In Vivo: Sulforaphane Is Protective in the Articular Joint." *Arthritis & Rheumatology* 65, no. 12 (December 2013): 3130–40.

Deshpande, Bhushan R., Jeffrey Katz, Daniel H. Solomon et al. "Number of Persons with Symptomatic Knee Osteoarthritis in the US: Impact of Race and Ethnicity, Age, Sex, and Obesity." *Arthritis Care & Research* 68, no. 12 (March 2016): 1743–50.

Fernández-Moreno, M., I. Rego, V. Carreira-Garcia, and F. J. Blanco. "Genetics in Osteoarthritis." *Current Genomics* 9, no. 8 (2008): 542–7.

Fontana, Robert J. "Acute Liver Failure Including Acetaminophen Overdose." *Medical Clinics of North America* 92, no. 4 (July 2008): 761–94, viii.

Gopalan, Ashwin, Sharon C. Reuben, Shamima Ahmed, Altaf S. Darvesh, Judit Hohmann, and Anupam Bishayee. "The Health Benefits of Blackcurrants." *Food & Function* 3, no. 8 (June 2012): 795–809.

Gorzynik-Debicka, Monika, Paulina Przychodzen, Francesco Cappello, et al. "Potential Health Benefits of Olive Oil and Plant Polyphenols." *International Journal of Molecular Sciences* 19, no. 3 (February 2018): 686.

Hashempur, M. H., Sarah Sadrneshin, Seyed Hamdollah Mosavat, and Alireza Ashraf. "Green Tea (*Camellia Sinensis*) for Patients with Knee Osteoarthritis: A Randomized Open-Label Active-Controlled Clinical Trial." *Clinical Nutrition* 37, no. 1 (February 2018): 85–90.

Hosseinzadeh, Azam, Davood Jafari, Tunku Kamarul, Abolfazll Bagheri, and Ali M. Sharifi. "Evaluating the Protective Effects and Mechanisms of Diallyl Disulfide on Interlukin-1β-Induced Oxidative Stress and Mitochondrial Apoptotic Signaling Pathways in Cultured Chondrocytes." *Journal of Cellular Biochemistry* 118, no. 7 (February 2017): 1879–88.

"Ibuprofen Drug Facts Label." US Food and Drug Administration. Last modified March 11, 2018. http://www.fda.gov/drugs/postmarket-drug-safety-information-patients-and-providers/ibuprofen-drug-facts-label.

John M. Eisenberg Center for Clinical Decisions and Communications Science. "Analgesics for Osteoarthritis." *Comparative Effectiveness Review Summary Guides for Clinicians*. Rockville, MD: Agency for Healthcare Research and Quality, 2012.

Knott, L., N. C. Avery, A. P. Hollander, and J. F. Tarlton. "Regulation of Osteoarthritis by Omega-3 (N-3) Polyunsaturated Fatty Acids in a Naturally Occurring Model of Disease." *Osteoarthritis and Cartilage* 19, no. 9 (September 2011): 1150–7.

Kompel, Andrew J., Frank W. Roemer, Akira M. Murakami, Luis E. Diaz, Michel D. Crema, and Ali Guermazi. "Intra-Articular Corticosteroid Injections in the Hip and Knee: Perhaps Not as Safe as We Thought?" *Radiology* 293, no. 3 (October 2019): 656–63.

Lee, H. S., C. H. Lee, H. C. Tsai, and Donald M. Salter. "Inhibition of Cyclooxygenase 2 Expression by Diallyl Sulfide on Joint Inflammation Induced by Urate Crystal and IL-1β." *Osteoarthritis and Cartilage* 17, no. 1 (2009): 91–9.

Lee, William M. "Acetaminophen and the US Acute Liver Failure Study Group: Lowering the Risks of Hepatic Failure." *Hepatology* 40, no. 1 (2004): 6–9.

Leong, Daniel J., Marwa Choudhury, Regina Hanstein, et al. "Green Tea Polyphenol Treatment Is Chondroprotective, Anti-Inflammatory, and

Palliative in a Mouse Post-Traumatic Osteoarthritis Model." *Arthritis Research & Therapy* 16, no. 6 (2014): 508.

Li, Yau, Jiaying Yao, Chunyan Han, et al. "Quercetin, Inflammation, and Immunity." *Nutrients* 8, no. 3 (2016): 167.

Lotz, Martin, and Virginia B. Kraus. "New Developments in Osteoarthritis. Posttraumatic Osteoarthritis: Pathogenesis and Pharmacological Treatment Options." *Arthritis Research & Therapy* 12, no. 3 (2010): 211.

Louie, Grant H., Maria G. Tektonidou, Alberto J. Caban-Martinez, and Michael M. Ward. "Sleep Disturbances in Adults with Arthritis: Prevalence, Mediators, and Subgroups at Greatest Risk. Data from the 2007 National Health Interview Survey." *Arthritis Care & Research* 63, no. 2 (2011): 247–60.

Mastaloudis, Angela, and Steve Wood. "Age-Related Changes in Cellular Protection, Purification, and Inflammation-Related Gene Expression: Role of Dietary Phytonutrients." *Annals of the New York Academy of Sciences* 1259, no. 1 (2012): 112–20.

Matsuno, Hiroaki, Hiroshi Nakamura, Kou Katayama, et al. "Effects of an Oral Administration of Glucosamine-Chondroitin-Quercetin Glucoside on the Synovial Fluid Properties in Patients with Osteoarthritis and Rheumatoid Arthritis." *Bioscience, Biotechnology, and Biochemistry* 73, no. 2 (2009): 288–92.

McDougall, Jason J., Milind M. Muley, Holly T. Philpott, et al. "Early Blockade of Joint Inflammation with a Fatty Acid Amide Hydrolase Inhibitor Decreases End-Stage Osteoarthritis Pain and Peripheral Neuropathy in Mice." *Arthritis Research & Therapy* 19, no. 1 (2017): 106.

Murphy, L. B., C. G. Helmick, T. A. Schwartz, et al. "One in Four People May Develop Symptomatic Hip Osteoarthritis in His or Her Lifetime." *Osteoarthritis Cartilage* 18, no. 11 (2010): 1372–9.

"Osteoarthritis." Accessed November 2019. my.clevelandclinic.org/health /diseases/5599-osteoarthritis-what-you-need-to-know.

"Osteoarthritis (OA)." Centers for Disease Control and Prevention. Last updated January 10, 2019. Accessed November 12, 2019. https://www.cdc.gov/arthritis/basics/osteoarthritis.htm.

"Osteoarthritis: Diagnosis and Treatment." Mayo Clinic. Last updated May 8, 2019. https://www.mayoclinic.org/diseases-conditions/osteoarthritis/diagnosis-treatment/drc-20351930.

Parkinson, Lisa, and Russell Keast. "Oleocanthal, a Phenolic Derived from Virgin Olive Oil: A Review of the Beneficial Effects on Inflammatory Disease." *International Journal of Molecular Sciences* 15, no. 7 (2014): 12323–34.

"Post-Traumatic Arthritis." Cleveland Clinic. Accessed November 12, 2019. https://my.clevelandclinic.org/health/diseases/14616-post-traumatic-arthritis.

Pottie, P., N. Presle, B. Terlain, P. Netter, D. Mainard, and F. Berenbaum. "Obesity and Osteoarthritis: More Complex Than Predicted!" *Annals of Rheumatic Diseases* 65, no. 11 (2006): 1403–5.

Qin, Jin, Kamil E. Barbour, Louise B. Murphy, et al. "Lifetime Risk of Symptomatic Hand Osteoarthritis: The Johnston County Osteoarthritis Project." *Arthritis & Rheumatology* 69, no. 6 (2017): 1204–12.

Schell, Jace, R. Hal Scofield, James R. Barrett, et al. "Strawberries Improve Pain and Inflammation in Obese Adults with Radiographic Evidence of Knee Osteoarthritis." *Nutrients* 9, no. 9 (2017).

Schumacher, H. Ralph, Sally Pullman-Mooar, Smita R. Gupta, et al. "Randomized Double-Blind Crossover Study of the Efficacy of a Tart Cherry Juice Blend in Treatment of Osteoarthritis (OA) of the Knee." *Osteoarthritis and Cartilage* 21, no. 8 (2013): 1035–41.

Segura-Carretero, Antonio, and José Antonio Curiel. "Current Disease-Targets for Oleocanthal as Promising Natural Therapeutic Agent." *International Journal of Molecular Sciences* 19, no. 10 (2018) 2899.

Sengupta, Krishanu, Krishnaraju V. Alluri, Andey Rama Satish, et al. "A Double Blind, Randomized, Placebo Controlled Study of the Efficacy and Safety of 5-Loxin® for Treatment of Osteoarthritis of the Knee." *Arthritis Research & Therapy* 10, no. 4 (2008): R85.

Siddiqui, Mahtab Z. "*Boswellia Serrata*, a Potential Antiinflammatory Agent: An Overview." *Indian Journal of Pharmaceutical Sciences* 73, no. 3 (2011): 255–61.

Simopoulos, Artemis. "The Importance of the Ratio of Omega-6/Omega-3 Essential Fatty Acids." *Biomedicine & Pharmacotherapy* 56, no. 8 (2002): 365–79.

Skrovankova, Sona, Daniela Sumczynski, Jiri Mlcek, Tunda Jurikova, and Jiri Sochor. "Bioactive Compounds and Antioxidant Activity in Different Types of Berries." *International Journal of Molecular Sciences* 16, no. 10 (2015): 24673–706.

Taylor, S. S., J. M. Hughes, C. J. Coffman, et al. "Prevalence of and Characteristics Associated with Insomnia and Obstructive Sleep Apnea among Veterans with Knee and Hip Osteoarthritis." *BMC Musculoskeletal Disorders* 19, no. 1 (2018): 79.

Thomas, Sally, Heather Browne, Ali Mobasheri, and Margaret P. Rayman. "What Is the Evidence for a Role for Diet and Nutrition in Osteoarthritis?" *Rheumatology* 57, supplement 4 (2018): iv61–iv74.

Villa-Forte, Alexandra. "Bones." *Merck Manuals Consumer Version.* Accessed December 21, 2019. https://www.merckmanuals.com/home/bone,-joint,-and-muscle-disorders/biology-of-the-musculoskeletal-system/bones.

Wollheim, Frank. "Early Stages of Osteoarthritis: the Search for Sensitive Predictors." *Annals of the Rheumatic Diseases* 62, no. 11 (2003): 1031–2.

INDEX

ACKNOWLEDGMENTS

I would like to thank my friends, family, and colleagues for supporting my writing dreams and goals. Also, thank you to the entire Callisto Media team for the seamless process of writing this incredible book.

ABOUT THE AUTHOR

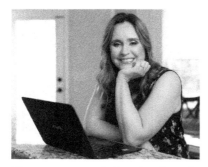

ANA REISDORF is a registered dietitian nutritionist with 13 years of experience in the field of nutrition and dietetics. Currently, she shares her passion on a larger scale as the founder of a health content agency. She is the author of two other books *The Lupus Cookbook* and *The Anti-Inflammatory Diet One-Pot Cookbook*. Ana lives in Nashville, Tennessee, with her husband and two boys. To learn more, visit her website at: www.anareisdorf.com.

Printed in the USA
CPSIA information can be obtained
at www.ICGtesting.com
CBHW040550110424
6562CB00013BA/6